DESIGN
YOUR LIFE

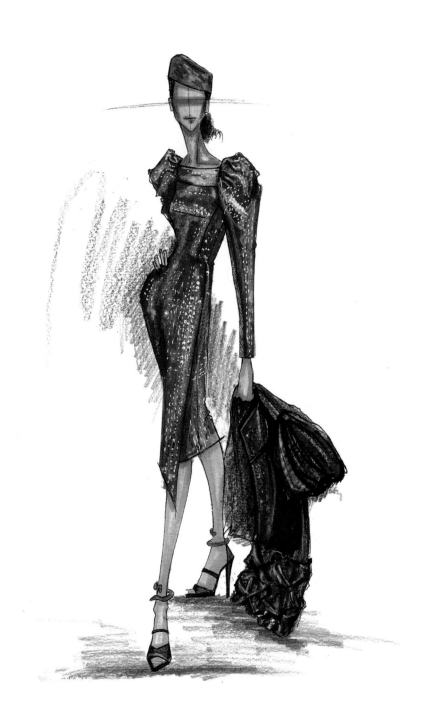

DESIGN YOUR LIFE

CREATING SUCCESS THROUGH PERSONAL STYLE

RACHEL ROY

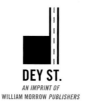

DEY ST.
AN IMPRINT OF
WILLIAM MORROW *PUBLISHERS*

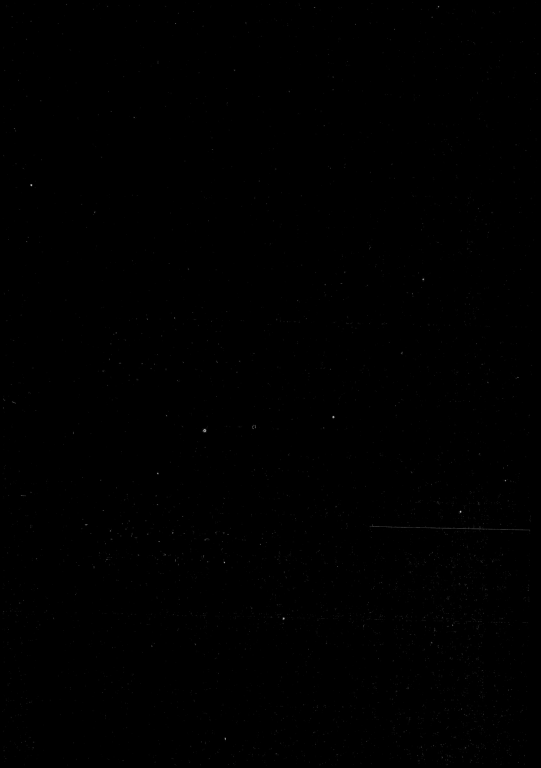

FOR MY DAUGHTERS.

YOU ARE NOT WHAT LIFE HANDS TO YOU,
YOU ARE THE LIFE YOU MAKE.

CONT

ENTS

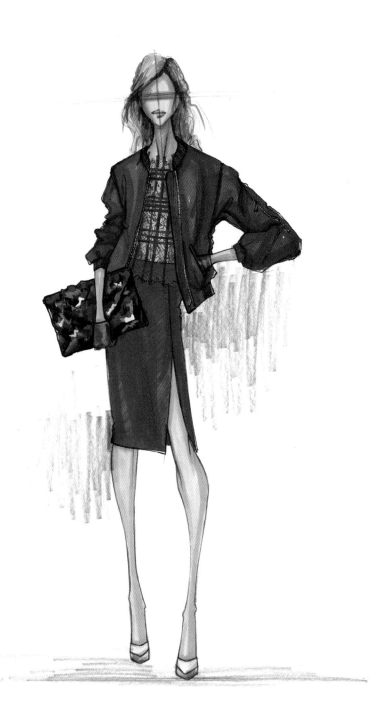

INTRODUCTION

Throughout the course of my life, I have learned some valuable lessons through both trial and error, as well as by surrounding myself with positive, strong people whom I admire. I am always excited by the opportunity to share what I have learned that has helped me grow, to share my story, and to pass along the tools that I use to design the life I want to live. I believe the tools have been presented to me so that I may pass them on to others to find the same peace or contentment.

I believe that in order to achieve the life you ultimately want, you have to embody the person living that life now.

There is so much we wish to accomplish, so much we place on ourselves to achieve, and what I know to be true is that every circumstance, every situation that has been put in front of us, is there to teach us something about the person we are meant to become. What I also know to be true is that we are in control of how we respond to each situation, therefore we create our lives based on *our* choices. The driving force of your life is you—not your parents, not your partner, not your friends. When we are young it is difficult to not blame our environment, so we settle into thinking things are happening *to* us instead of *for* us. But the complete opposite is actually true. Our experiences are uniquely ours, presented to guide us to become the people we are meant to be, to live our truest versions of ourselves. And our choices matter. So, the minute you make a choice, really make a choice, own it and commit to it, you are on a whole new level of existence. This applies to every aspect of your life, from professional to personal. Your choices are yours to make. What career you pursue, where you choose to spend your time, what you choose to spend your time doing, and who you choose to spend your time with. What you choose to wear, how you choose to speak to people, how you choose to carry yourself, how you choose to react. All your choice.

————

Which brings us to designing the life you want. To do so, first you need more than a vague idea or a distant dream. It starts with dreaming, yes, but it also takes planning, creating, and above all, harnessing the universe to turn your dreams into reality. In this book, I will share my own journey from young woman to mother of two and successful entrepreneur. I hope that my story will encourage you to identify your dream in life and help you recognize your own personal path to success through what brings you joy. I will share how my experiences working in the fashion industry taught me to choose to dress in a manner that helped me to achieve my dreams, and how you can do the same with whatever it is you wish to pursue.

Clothing and personal style can affect how you feel about yourself and therefore how you treat yourself, so for me, fashion plays a major role in self-esteem and the type of energy I give out.

Self-respect, self-love, self-rule. It's all in how we take control of choices in our lives from simple to immense. What we can accomplish when we feel happy and whole is astonishing. The universe plans more for us than we can even dream up. But to live up to our potential, to be able to see it through, we must show up aware, confident, and joy-filled; that's the catch.

––––––––––

Throughout the course of my journey, fashion and style have made a vital contribution each step along the way. I hope that my personal stories will help inspire you to make imaginative and effective fashion choices that can help your own aspirations become a reality. My goal and intent is to advocate focusing on the person you want to be and making choices based on where you want to go, in order to get the job you aspire to have. This book is written for the person who knows she has a destiny but may need a little help creating the life she's always imagined having. I will illustrate how the daughter of a carpenter, who only owned a single pair of sneakers growing up, became the leader of a fashion company.

I wholeheartedly believe that you get back what you put into the universe, and that the law of attraction plays an essential role in your life path. But I also believe in what I call the law of intention. How do you intend to be received? How do you set your intention for the day?

I believe it starts in the morning when you're brushing your teeth, saying your sun salutations, or in my case preparing hot water with lemon. Before I check my calendar and go over the details of my day, I send a prayer of thankfulness for at least five things I am grateful for. Positive thoughts beget positive outcomes, and for me this involves thinking of ways to activate myself to be as productive as I can be on any given day. I also do something as simple as choose one person a morning to send a positive e-mail to. It may surprise you the peace it passes as well as the peace that comes back to you when you do.

Beyond that, what is my greater intention? I want to be a guiding light to my daughters. I want to continue to work hard and be passionate about what I do. I want to create designs that make women feel strong and beautiful. I want to help women find their voice. All of these internal intentions can be reflected on my exterior. Part of the beauty of being a woman is being able to express our feelings through fashion so easily; with shape, color, texture, and style. We do better when we look better because we feel better.

I keep a small sign in my kitchen and another in my office that reads: "What Good Shall I Do This Day?" I want my actions to improve daily in terms of business, household, and health, sure, but I also want to put goodness back into the world, even if that merely means smiling at a stranger or setting my unread e-mails aside to take time to organize health and spirit into my day.

In the following chapters I will introduce you to my favorite signature pieces and my invaluable "uniform" staples that help me quickly feel the way I need to in order to be a productive soul; items from my collections over the years as well as those that I've admired from others. I'll explain the inspiration behind specific creations, the effectiveness of certain garments, and the personal and aesthetic philosophies they embody.

When I was first starting out in the fashion industry I worked in the mailroom of a major clothing company. Even though it would be tough to gain any notice in that position, I made the conscious decision not to show up in casual or poorly made clothes in which to sort mail all day. Instead, I dressed like I was about to self-promote to CEO. Why? Not because I set out to take anyone's job, but rather, it was twofold. First, I felt better when I looked better, and for me looking better meant feeling polished and put together. Second, although I knew that I was fit for a higher position, I needed others to realize this as well. So I dressed the part. I also paid attention to my surroundings; I knew the company I was working for needed leadership, as all companies do. I also knew my strengths and my weaknesses. (That awareness is key. Knowing what you are not good at is just as important as knowing where you excel.) I excelled at design and I excelled at staying focused and finishing a project and organizing a story into a collection of clothing. Staying focused on what type of career I wanted and had a passion for gave me the confidence to say what was needed to create a successful women's and children's brand extension at a company that made only men's clothing at the time. I had always observed that those who don't speak up miss out. But I would add to that: when you do speak up, make sure you have something of value to offer. Don't just ask questions; offer solutions. And most important, make yourself needed in the areas in which you excel. Offer to help in situations where you see help is needed rather than waiting to be asked. Years later, when I was promoted to creative director of women's within that company, I continued to set the bar higher for myself; I created designs that I wanted to wear myself and offered them to the partners as a brand extension. When the owners turned me down, I was slightly disappointed at first, but I just took my designs elsewhere and created my own brand with the once rejected samples. A buyer at Bergdorf Goodman saw me wearing my designs in a lifestyle photograph in *Women's Wear Daily,* found my number, called me, and wrote my first order. Not stopping at the first, second, or third rejection is essential to life in general. Eventually, I was the creator and owner of my own company, with designs that represented my point of view. Throughout the seven years it took me to go from the mailroom to creative director, and the fourteen years working in retail stores prior to that, I kept dressing the part until I had the part, until it was just an element of my everyday life. It's something that every woman has it in her to do. If I could do it, you can do it. The very fact that you're here with me now tells me that you have the intention. And that is the first step.

It's not just about convincing others to believe in you; it's about convincing yourself to believe in you, too. Where do you intend to go, and how will you get there? Looking like the most put-together, elegant, responsible, knowing version of yourself makes you feel and act as such—someone that any person would look at and say, "That woman is someone I would like to know more about." If you don't look like you believe in you, why should anyone else? There are certainly days when I don't feel like the best version of me. It's incredible how quickly that moody moment can be quelled by tucking myself into a chic, feel-good trench dress and painting on a bold lip. Walk taller, feel taller. It works every time!

Dressing this way doesn't mean you have to resort to fancy labels and expensive handbags. Sharp lines, a sophisticated structure, and pieces that fit your frame without wrinkles and frays; that's what makes you look and feel strong. If you aim to be sleek and sharp minded, choose sharp and sleek lines in your clothing. Same goes for romantic and mysterious. Powerful and intelligent. Dress for the mood you would like to be in or the element you wish to represent.

When I design for a woman, I'm designing an idea that will take her to the next level in any capacity. I want what she's wearing to help her achieve her dream job—even create one if the right opportunity isn't out there. Give her a sense that her joie de vivre shines so brightly she could stop traffic. Encourage her to be a little bolder in her decision-making. Emit good energy, certainty, and joy—that's what I want my clothes to do for me.

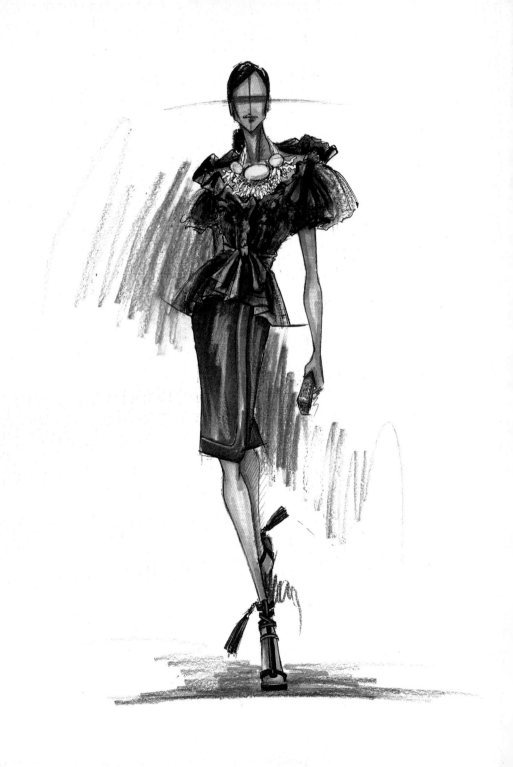

· 1 ·

LETTING YOUR DREAMS LEAD IN FASHION AND IN LIFE

I've learned that you shouldn't go through life with a catcher's mitt on both hands; you need to be able to throw something back.

—MAYA ANGELOU

I began designing my life a long time ago, although I didn't realize it at the time.

The U-shaped peninsula where I grew up in Northern California had two sides separated by more than just water. Facing the west were affluent cities like Monterey, Carmel, and Pebble Beach. Facing east was a low-income community, Seaside.

That's where my family lived. My mother was a Dutch computer programmer and my father a college professor who had emigrated from India. A self-taught carpenter as well, my father knocked out the walls along the back of our house and replaced them with floor-to-ceiling windows he found at construction sites or city dumps to let in the views overlooking the Pacific Ocean. The mesmerizing panorama was a constant reminder that although we lived on the less well-off side of town, both sides of the divide had access to the same picturesque views of the water. This implicit equality instilled some strong convictions in my mind and in my heart. For several different reasons I grew up with the inherent belief that all people are equal, no matter the level of income, status in society, or skin color. This firm faith in fair and equal rights, coupled with my father's pride in his roots, taught me to understand and appreciate the beauty of being biracial. Having the opportunity to learn about and connect to both my father's Indian side and my mother's Dutch heritage has always felt like a privilege rather than a burden. My biracial identity has been an advantage and a key in shaping a solid self-identity, not a hindrance.

The ocean divide that I woke up with and went to sleep with for seventeen years was also a constant reminder that there was a better life out there somewhere in the world, beyond Seaside. I came to see the expansive ocean view as a symbolic representation of all the opportunities and possibilities that existed outside of our microcosm. I was always grateful for the blessings we did have, which I knew were far more plentiful than what others in our community had, or what most had in the impoverished cities of India, yet my gratitude did not impede my curiosity. I knew there was more for myself and for my brother and for any one of my friends who wanted a life they dreamed about. For me old movies provided that knowledge of escape.

Growing up, I was only allowed to watch black-and-white films from the 1930s through the 1950s or documentaries on animals and nature. To this day, my coffee table is a perfect reflection of my varied tastes, piled high with issues of both *National Geographic* and *Vogue*. My early immersion in vintage films and the art of nature greatly influenced my designs and personal style. Screen sirens such as Ava Gardner and Tallulah Bankhead opened my eyes to wardrobe foundation staples that were feminine and classic, soft but strong. Clothing was structured to a T and tailored to fit like a glove.

12

Although the pieces rarely showed much skin, they were cinched and taut, and showcased each woman's curvaceous shape. One of the aspects I loved about those old films was that women were allowed and encouraged to be equal parts strong and sexy. As a young girl, I was able to recognize the power in presenting and projecting sophistication, elegance, and a healthy dose of sensuality, blended with having something to say. I knew having an opinion that stood for something mattered, at least in those old films that my father had me watch. In those films the heroines were honored for being smart.

From my side of town, sitting in our weathered but well-kept house, I would look out of the window walls and imagine that the affluent people on the other side of the peninsula were living the glamorous lives I saw depicted in the old movies. My childhood journals are filled with sketches of the beautiful, refined, alluring clothes and accessories I dreamt about, all inspired by those legendary screen goddesses. As I got older, my imagination grew more vivid and focused, and I began creating my own magazines, meticulously designing each cover in what I believed to be the sophisticated style I'd come to admire. Luckily, my sweet mother had the foresight and penchant for sentimental keepsakes to save this early collection of homemade periodicals, and she shared the mint-condition magazines with me as I set out to start my own collection. I didn't consciously know what I was doing at the time, but in retrospect I realize that I was designing the life I truly wanted and hoped to one day live. I was setting my intentions visually.

THE CREATION

I have an ongoing love affair with the juxtaposition of masculine and feminine ideals. I blame Old Hollywood, and my obsession with those classic films from my childhood, for my enduring fascination with contrasting and complementary traits. The fashion of the 1940s has always been my greatest inspiration, from a time when women were praised for being ultrafeminine but undeniably strapping at once. The styles of the era encouraged women to be simultaneously assertive yet alluring, such a modern sensibility—it's that mind-set that inspires my adoration for a timeless piece that I firmly believe can transform any outfit, wardrobe, and overall aesthetic: the well-tailored blazer. In this case I will play favorites—it is one of the most important items in a woman's closet.

14

Throughout my entire adult life, I've felt the pull to find that perfect blazer, a piece of clothing that, when paired with a slinky dress or a low-cut V-neck, completely exemplifies the kind of life I always imagined my screen sirens living in their off time. It's incredible what strength a fitted blazer can lend to an outfit. Pulling it over a pair of distressed jeans instantly upgrades an otherwise casual ensemble to a higher level of existence. Adding it on top of a silk cocktail dress infuses an otherwise soft, delicate look with confidence and authority. I have been awed and inspired by that juxtaposition of soft and strong for as long as I can remember.

I'd always felt no other item of clothing could rival the brilliance of a blazer; however, the immensely pulled-together-looking topper comes in at a close second. A topper is a trench coat meets cardigan

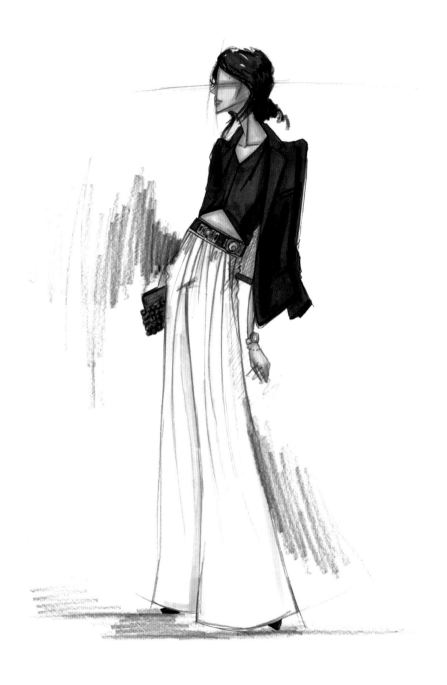

meets blazer, all rolled into one. In other words, the ideal wardrobe staple. Usually made from woven fabric, much like the blazer, the topper can also come in softer fabrics such as a knit. In the 1950s, Grace Kelly would have called it her car coat. This sophisticated piece drapes demurely over the shoulders and loosely falls over the frame, typically hitting mid-thigh. The sleeves can be short and worn over a long-sleeved blouse or they can be long to the wrist. Toppers are formal in spirit, more polished than a cardigan, yet less grandiose than a cape. But no matter where it falls on the extravagance scale, this classic item is a true style saver. I'd consider the woman who reaches for a topper to be an outside-the-box thinker who is confident, creative, and self-assured enough to not feel the need to wear something tight to be noticed. I own toppers in stripes, florals, and fantastic storytelling prints like palm trees. I can assure you I get a ton of mileage out of these iconic pieces. In addition to their versatility and simplicity, I admire how they are a true representation of the sophistication of my favorite fashion era.

THE INSPIRATION

When I was younger, just beginning to open my eyes to the world I lived in, I started my own vision boards—even if at the time, I only thought of it as doodling and cutting up magazines. And to this day, creating and maintaining a vision board is something I still do on a monthly basis. Having inspiring images to gaze at throughout the day keeps me on track and accountable, continuously motivating me to embody the woman I aspire to be and to not forget the things I strive to become in the day-to-day whirlwinds and diversions that happen in life.

The purpose of a vision board is to inspire you, to cultivate your tastes, and to give you a concrete goal to work toward every day. Constructing and displaying a vision board is about calling certain things into your life, and having the constant visual reminder of your aspirations right in front of you is hugely motivating. Otherwise known as the law of attraction, the act of invoking and inviting your coveted desires into your life is an incredibly powerful tool. Designers often use vision boards as guidance down a tunnel of thought or as a way to dream up a story that can translate into a cohesive collection.

When I was about five or six, I would spend my free time cutting out images from magazines I found throughout the house or

17

at the college my father worked for. I would, painstakingly, artfully arrange the cutouts to display the narrative I wanted to get across in the most beautiful way. And I came to find out that whatever you spend your time thinking about and looking at *will* show up in your life. I observed it in my own experiences, and I've seen it materialize for others around me. If you are drawn to or inspired by an image in the back of *Vogue* of a capable woman who looks like she's all business, clip it to your board. If something in you melts when you look at a hippie-chic hottie with loose waves in her hair, clip that to your board. Images of flowers, a type of cuisine, architecture, and so on—whatever it is, if it tugs at your heartstrings, it's meant to be on your board. It doesn't have to be logical or rational; in fact, sometimes it's more meaningful if it just speaks to your subconscious, or soul. This is how you discover what you want to call into your life; simply things that make you happy. It should be something that feels familiar when you look at it, even though you can't explain why. It feels like you want to know more, or in some cases, it just seems *right*. Your subconscious is there to guide you each and every time, and all it requires is paying attention and perceiving the way that certain environments, images, people, situations, colors, sounds, etc., make you feel. It might not make sense in the moment. It might not make sense ever. But this is how the universe speaks to you. What else could it be? Be still and listen.

This is your place to put a visual representation of whatever it is you desire, to have one beautiful corner of the world filled with things that inspire you to be the best version of you, to live the life you want to create.

After living in New York for almost twenty years and considering a home in California, I was first drawn to architectural magazines and did not understand this sudden push for magazines that featured homes only and no fashion, until after weeks of pulling the same image in different settings, it was clear: I longed for a different environment; I longed to live by the sea. Clipping pictures of beautiful views of the ocean or the gorgeous gardens of Tuscany and Florence, the kinds of things that I wanted more of in my own world, eventually enabled me to recognize and realize my dream. I now reside in California with my two daughters with a beautiful garden and a pool; next stop, the ocean! As the universe would have it, once I moved to California I met my now business partners. Everything happens for a reason and it starts with a call, an urge, a longing from your soul for action toward that which moves your heart. I remember clipping out a gorgeous image of the interior of an airplane—in retrospect I believe it was a sign that I was ready to take flight, to take a giant leap into the next part of my life, perhaps? Let the images speak to you and guide you. Choose with your heart, not your head, and they will make sense to you as time goes on.

Now that I'm living happily in California, I have actually used some of the images from that original board to inspire the décor of my home. It feels empowering and gives reason to that inner voice, my subconscious, to have taken the things that spoke to me and see them actualized in my real life. I was designing my life—not the one I was living at the time, but the one I was hoping to live.

I can't emphasize enough how important it is to allow the vision board to be a haven of creativity and wishful thinking—the images you include needn't be realistic or plausible. To this day, most of the things I put on my vision board are things that I haven't achieved or actualized yet, but that I want to call into my own life. For example, that ocean-view home is still a dream I'm following. I have a bushel of photos of houses overlooking the sea, and while I don't have one of my own yet, I know that I will. Experiencing the magic and miracles inherent in the vision board has taught me to stop questioning and doubting, and to start trusting myself.

For a very long time, I have had a photo of Cary Grant prominently displayed on my board—one from a formal time period, long gone, when men used to wear suits even for the most casual event. He looks like someone I'd want to have a conversation with—what book is he reading? What wine does he drink? What journey is he headed off on? What does he think and feel? The simple photograph evokes so many thoughts and feelings that I can't help but be drawn to it. Its outward simplicity masks a complexity that I find so compelling, it's kept my attention for years.

It's no secret now that I've always been inspired by men's details in women's clothing, and this photo of Grant constantly reminds me that a touch of formality can elevate any moment. Even if it's a Saturday and I'm not re-quired to look particularly dressy, I will put on some style of a jacket or blazer to elevate my outfit and my assurance. The way I feel when I look at Grant in the photo is the exact emotion I would like to evoke in people when they look at me. Looking at Grant inspires me to put a little extra effort into projecting a dignified, pulled-together presentation, and to always look ahead, with curiosity, at what I may learn each day.

THE PHILOSOPHY

I often feel the right clothing, whether it's a perfect blazer, a graceful topper, or an eye-catching accessory, can elevate me into the world I wish to inhabit. My vision board and the dashing image of Cary Grant remind me of that every day. I determined early on that I'm a completely visual person—I process and retain information best when I have images to accompany the ideas. When I have visual cues in plain sight, I'm less likely to forget the intentions they rep-resent. The tried-and-true saying "out of sight, out of mind" is a philosophy that unfortunately does not escape me. I know I can get caught up in the day-to-day rush of life and forget the details that make me creative, inspired, driven, and passionate. Surrounding myself with concrete images keeps my priorities at the top of my mind. I am not alone in this—I believe most people respond best to visuals, even if they view the world in black and white. Everyone has things that make their heart sing, and looking at those ideas as clippings every day will call them into their lives.

21

Starting your own vision board will help you begin to identify your personal style. Not everybody can spend hours reading fashion blogs or afford the latest in designer clothing. But the inability to invest in these areas in the present moment doesn't mean you can't curate your outward appearance to the world and create a spirit that you hope will manifest in everything you hope to achieve. Whether you tend toward Zara staples or Chanel couture, the choices you make in how you present yourself to the world have a huge impact on your self-image. Once you identify your own personal style, you will start to get a sense not only of how you currently feel about yourself and your present life, but of how you wish to feel about yourself and the world around you. Don't underestimate the power of presentation: by dressing and embodying the values and aspirations you truly connect to, you are setting a goal of becoming more like the person you're building on that vision board in front of you. The vision board version of you *is* you—the difference is that she has all the certainty we sometimes lack (we all occasionally fail at feeling extraordinary—it's par for the course for most of us to slip). Starting to dress like her is not just a stylistic choice: dressing the part means embodying her poise and unshakable faith in her values. It means starting to walk and talk like her as a way to channel that crucial confidence. The results will be almost immediate: the people around you will sense the shift in your energy and respond positively because you will believe it yourself. The laws of attraction meet the laws of intention. You are believing your best "you" into existence.

As you can see, the vision board is a powerful tool that can inspire you in a million different ways. I'm surrounded by them on a daily basis both personally and professionally.

Keep this in mind—when you look at colors and images on your board, how do they make you feel? Lemon yellow, sunny? Grass green, fresh and breezy? Or gray and muddled, like a dark storm cloud? Jealous, competitive, or depressed? If an image somehow fills you with shame or self-doubt, it should not make it to the board. Am I sidetracked by a model's washboard stomach, does it make me feel badly about my own midsection, or does it inspire me? If it does anything negative to my energy, it doesn't belong on my vision board. This is an inspiration-only zone, and I have to be completely candid with myself about what the images do to my self-esteem, sense of self-worth, and motivation to achieve what's best for me. In order for the vision board to truly help you achieve your goals and not hinder your progress, be honest with yourself and ensure that the clippings you choose do not lead you down a critical path of judgment, but instead take you through a progressive journey of self-discovery.

There is an image currently on my board of a model in jeans, a strong-shouldered red blazer, and a crisp shirt. The classic red blazer is slung casually over her shoulders. She is walking her formidable dog, who is sporting a natural rope leash. And most important, her subtle smile radiates an inner poise and peace that I find magnetic. It's these nuances about her that I like and feel drawn to—so natural, simple, and effortless with her style. She's an individual even though she's classically dressed, and her inner beauty effectively shines through because it's clear she feels comfortable not only in her clothes, but in her skin. That is what inspires me. What is the entire story saying from the image? These are questions you can ask yourself as you guide yourself to understanding your style and how you personally want to design your life through the images you choose.

Your vision board can help you figure out how to work with what you already own. We can all work with what we have and find clothes that flatter us and make us feel like the best versions of ourselves without breaking the bank. I always start by going into my closet to find the pieces of clothing that speak to the woman I'd like to portray. Whether it's for a meeting next Monday morning, or for a date this Thursday night, I'll find a couple of pieces I haven't worn in a while and figure out a new way to make them work for me. This exercise helps me make a shift and evolve my style while allowing some of my familiar pieces to see the light of day. It doesn't require a shopping spree, a major splurge, or even a major time investment. All it takes is some thoughtfulness and creativity about the style and persona I want to cultivate.

I suggest that you take what's you, in your closet and in your life, and modernize it, add onto it, make it work for the you you've always wanted to be. Don't let preconceived notions about who you should be or who you've always been cloud your judgment: just let the ideal you shine through and guide your choices. Your vision board is your inspiration, to start highlighting your best attributes, and to breathe new life into your old pieces to create the best you possible. Design

LETTING YOUR DREAMS LEAD IN FASHION AND IN LIFE

your new life, the one you're aspiring toward, not the one you're escaping. As Emerson said, don't be pushed by your problems; be led by your dreams. Be comfortable, be confident. But above all, be you.

Creating Your Vision Board:

Whether you cut it up, rip it out, or copy and click is up to you. I am all for creating digital vision boards as well as paper. I keep several boards on Pinterest to inspire my style, home décor, recipes, floral arrangements, and so on. Warning: once you start it's very difficult to stop!

No rhyme or reason. If you love it, use it. It might not make sense to you now but at some point in the future you'll understand why you were so drawn to certain images. This has happened to me time and time again. Follow your heart and listen to the inner voice; it knows what your passion is.

Set the mood. Create an atmosphere that is conducive to hearing your inner voice. I like to light candles, listen to music, and enjoy the process.

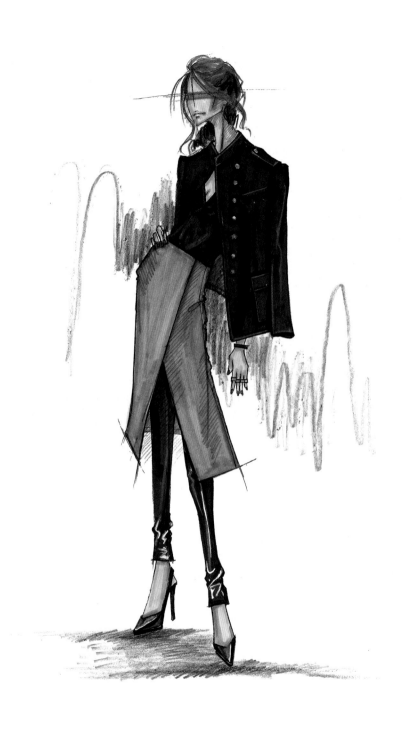

GENDER JUXTAPOSITION

MIXING MASCULINE AND FEMININE FOR A LOOK THAT IS POISED AND POWERFUL

We try to convince
ourselves that
somehow doing it all
is a badge of honor,
but for many of us
it is a necessity, and
we have to be very
careful not to
lose ourselves
in the process.

—FIRST LADY MICHELLE OBAMA

Being a fashion-loving, style-conscious high-school student with only one pair of sneakers wasn't very easy, fun, or inspiring. Quite frankly, it was just embarrassing. The single pair of light gray Keds-knockoff sneakers I bought at Payless were for both gym class and my everyday life. We couldn't afford new clothes to fit my sprouting frame or my burgeoning dreams, and everything I owned had to be multifunctional—style wasn't really a factor.

While my mother was always innately graceful and quietly elegant, her wardrobe wasn't exactly enviable, so instead I usually opted for my father's hand-me-downs. His men's Levi's 501 jeans were just long enough to fit me then, and it might be a surprise to hear but they're still my favorite today. When my dad was just fourteen, his parents insisted he leave home and go work for the Indian Navy. His life-altering move had a somewhat unexpected impact on his future daughter's wardrobe. Luckily for me, he saved all of his sailor jackets, and well before it was on-trend to incorporate military-style pieces into everyday outfits, I was wearing the decorative-patch heavy wool, box-frame fitting navy jackets with my hand-me-down cream Levi's. I had zero money but because I had vision, imagination, and a healthy dose of ingenuity, I had something else that came to be much more important. When it came to style, I was rich in that department.

Today, menswear remains a constant, if not a main theme of my collections, although from a distance one might not be able to tell. While masculine pieces have been appropriated by fashion-forward females for decades, menswear has more recently emerged as a mainstream trend favored by women throughout the world. It's also one of the secret ingredients that make the well-dressed women behind the scenes in the fashion industry look so spectacular. These innovators run the brands that we all covet, and they know that a tuxedo pant paired with a brilliant heel is a tried-and-true way to define a chic personal uniform staple. They can throw a well-tailored coat or blazer over just about anything, and instantly look dignified, effortless, and in control. They know that these traditionally masculine pieces mixed with a feminine silhouette create a fresh, sexy, prestigious look that speaks volumes to one's character. The seemingly opposing forces actually blend beautifully on the body, and the combination complements just about any size and shape. It's no secret that I love contradictions in fashion, whether it's neutrals versus bold colors, or prints set against other, incongruous patterns. By blending the masculine and feminine, the edgy aesthetic plays perfectly against the softer cuts and curves, creating a brand-new style from two familiar fashion worlds.

THE CREATION

One of the first pieces I ever designed was a truly classic wardrobe staple: the trench coat dress. I was attracted to the trench because of its flattering silhouette and reflection of both strength and femininity. Since there already were so many iterations of the iconic piece, however, it was important for me to make my own creation completely unique yet functional. To add edginess to an otherwise very classic look, I decided to construct the details of the coat out of black leather. Though I added a modern fabric embellishment to the mix, I kept the shape traditional with a double-breasted top. Along the skirt of the trench, I designed the leather into circular, patterned laser cutouts reaching from the hem to high up the leg. A layer of organza was sewn in underneath to give just a hint of sheer, translucent protection in order to reveal a bit of the wearer's legs as she moved. The thought behind the overall design was completely calculated; I like the notion of a woman being strategically inviting, looking demure yet classic at the same time.

My version of the trench coat gave women an experience. It wasn't merely a jacket or a coat, but was actually also intended to serve double duty as a dress. The classic shape created an elongated effect and slenderized, allowing the wearer to convey a pulled-together sensibility with no distractions. The leather cutouts introduced an element of strength mixed with sex appeal, and the finished product was a piece I felt reflected a beautiful, classic yet modern combination that never goes out of style.

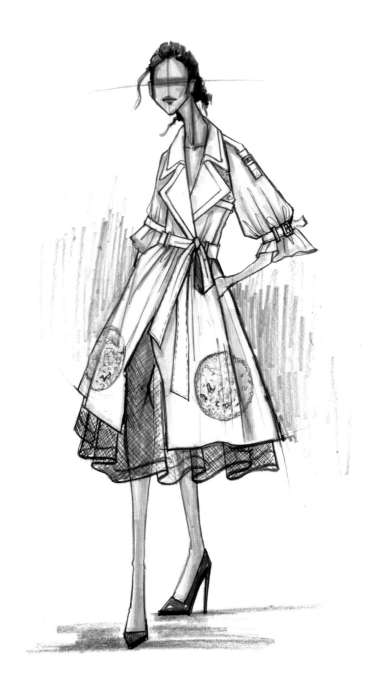

THE INSPIRATION

The trench coat has been an important piece in my fashion evolution. When I was in high school, wearing out my dad's 501s, the one item in my mother's closet that I truly coveted was her camel trench coat, which came paired with a brown faux snakeskin belt. Although we didn't lead a life of luxury—far from it, in fact—when she wore that elegant trench coat, she seemed to transform into her version of Grace Kelly. I loved watching my mother sit at her tiny armoire and apply her Oil of Olay. She'd put on her makeup with her final touch always being a spritz of Chanel No. 5. It was her daily prework routine, and I found the ritual fascinating. The finishing touch was what stood out to me above the rest: I observed that when she pulled out her camel trench coat for the day, she stood up a bit taller; she moved with an ease that only the most graceful and confident have. Although my mother's innate beauty always shone through despite our humble lifestyle, none of her other outfits gave her the same air of regality as that trench did.

This lesson that confidence can stem from what you are wearing and how it makes you feel is something I learned early on, and that notion is what inspires me as a designer today. It brings me indescribable joy and fulfillment to know that I am designing something for women to empower them to feel strong and sexy, even on days they perhaps woke up feeling otherwise. When I'm at the office, it is my role to lead and inspire the team, and it is critical that I convey the message of strength, intelligence, and purpose as consistently as I can. The way I successfully achieve this is by purposely wearing clothes and accessories that represent and embody those qualities. If I showed up to the office looking weak and unkempt, it would set the tone not only for me, but for those looking to me for guidance and inspiration. Wearing an elegant, sharp outfit motivates me, as well as those who work for me, to be smart and structured in our professional lives.

That said, menswear is by no means limited to professional settings; borrowing from the boys is a fabulous way to stand out at any function. Some of my favorite go-to pieces are meant for a man yet tailored specifically for me. Accessories such as a bow tie or a cummerbund are a fun way to man up an outfit, and a good way to infuse a familiar outfit with fresh details. I also love a tie over a fitted white collar button-down, and I regularly wear a tuxedo jacket over skirts or fitted trousers, which I consider to be the perfect day-to-night ensemble. The common rule of thumb governing all these looks is the principle of balance. Going head to toe in a masculine look would be overkill for me. But incorporating menswear pieces while staying mindful of your frame and curves, and allowing room for some feminine flourishes, is the perfect way to wear menswear styles.

34

THE PHILOSOPHY

In the late 1800s, women were unable to ride bicycles due to their voluminous, floor-sweeping skirts. Anything shorter, tighter, or more practical (in other words, anything that would have actually allowed a woman the freedom of motion necessary to ride a bike), was deemed promiscuous-looking. Bicycles were for men and boys only, and women and girls were left observing. Over the years, fashion slowly adapted with the times, and bicycle costumes were eventually designed in order to allow women to 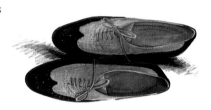 preserve their modesty while enabling them to safely ride a bicycle. Thankfully, we have come a long way since then, but when you reflect, those times really weren't so long ago. While it can be easy to take our fashion freedoms for granted these days, women of the not-so-distant past were obligated to fall in line with style standards that often restricted and limited their abilities to move through the world. Today, I embrace the opportunity to wear trousers, men's shirts, and oxford shoes simply because I like how effortless and becoming they look on a woman, and I am grateful that I have the freedom to choose when and how I want to incorporate these pieces. To me those choices also represent being able to have freedom of choice in every aspect of my life, including the office. I will never restrict myself with rules about what I can and cannot wear to work, in the same manner that I will never restrict myself in terms of what I can and cannot accomplish. We must set our standards according to the goals we have for ourselves—many of which can be discovered through our vision boards if we are uncertain. A full life is one lived on your own terms, with your own rules the key to better understanding what those terms are and mean to you.

As a designer, it is my continual objective to create stylish outfits for women that promote confidence and self-esteem. By dressing

35

like the supreme, sharp, self-assured woman you aspire to be, you are motivating and empowering yourself to actually become that woman. To help you build your own arsenal of masculine wardrobe staples, I've created a list of key menswear-inspired pieces that I believe every woman should have in her closet. The goal when trying menswear is to incorporate one or two masculine elements into your outfit that actually accentuate your femininity. For the right balance, I always throw in at least one feminine touch, such as spikey, pointy heels or a brightly colored accessory. Even something as simple as finishing the look off with a bold lipstick exudes femininity.

———

KEY MENSWEAR PIECES EVERY WOMAN SHOULD HAVE

THE CLASSIC OXFORD SHIRT

My body image wasn't at its best when I returned to work after giving birth to my daughter Tallulah. The idea of looking polished and put together seemed a lifetime away and entirely impossible. The oxford shirt did for me what it has done and continues to do for many women: it camouflaged problem areas while giving me a boost of confidence in my body. I believe any woman can feel beautiful in an oxford shirt, no matter her bra size, what her waistline looks like, what her hip shape is, or how she perceives any other area of her body that might not be as perfect as she'd like it to be. Like a bathing suit cover-up, the oxford shirt is a universal item that can conceal the places that make us cringe. If my kids want a beach day and I'm not exactly feeling like wearing a bathing suit in public, I'll don a beautiful cover-up and just go with it. I can't miss out on fun activities and time with my children just because I'm feeling insecure about my body, and I hate to think there are women out there missing out on their lives because their self-doubts about their bodies are holding them back. Covering up doesn't have to mean hiding beneath a too-big blouse or running errands in an unflattering, oversized sweater on days like this. The oxford can be the one item in your closet that will boost your certainty no matter what your body shape is, and can effectively enhance your figure while keeping the parts you're not so thrilled about under wraps.

This classic button-down is your wardrobe's best friend, adding just the right amount of sophistication to any outfit. The oxford is also incredibly versatile, made from an endless array of fabrics to choose from, as well as a variety of colors, prints, and patterns. Play with the various styles until you find your signature, but be sure to have at least one solid, crispy white top in the mix. I am all for branching out to cropped, boxy, and tuxedo styles, but having at least one basic white button-down shirt in a traditional structure is paramount. An important detail I both incorporate into my designs and look out for when filling my closet is button placement. I like my oxford shirts to have a button situated directly under my bra, so that when the outfit calls for a low, unbuttoned look, like it did with my

Tip: When mixing prints or playing with color blocking, allow the loud pieces to compete, yet ground them with a solid button-down shirt.

men's tuxedo, it shows just the right amount of skin based on button placement. Otherwise, if the button placement opens directly at the bra, you will never be able to achieve the low-cut look that many masculine suits require.

Not only is the oxford shirt wearable in every season, but it also successfully transitions to all of your roles. My favorite professional look is a buttoned-up shirt tucked into tailored trousers or a textured pencil skirt. When I'm going for something more casual, I like to add a cardigan or blazer thrown over the shoulders. You can seamlessly go from a conference to cocktails without an outfit change by simply rolling up the sleeves, undoing a few buttons, and adding a darker lip. When running errands or shuttling my girls around, the key to casual sophistication is pairing boyfriend jeans, a cotton A-line skirt, or loose shorts with an oxford.

THE GOES-WITH-EVERYTHING BLAZER

The piece that will most transform the garments in your closet will always be the blazer. Not only does it instantly upgrade any outfit, but it also downsizes your shape. In my opinion, you cannot have enough well-fitting blazers. This must-have closet staple actually has quite a significant history. Blazers earned an important reputation in playing a part in the women's movement, establishing equality and position for both genders in the workplace. But back then, we were just ap-

Tip: Don't limit yourself to traditional patterns or colors. After you have your classic colors in check, expand to your favorite print or pattern. For me, it is gold sailor stripe ribbons at the sleeve.

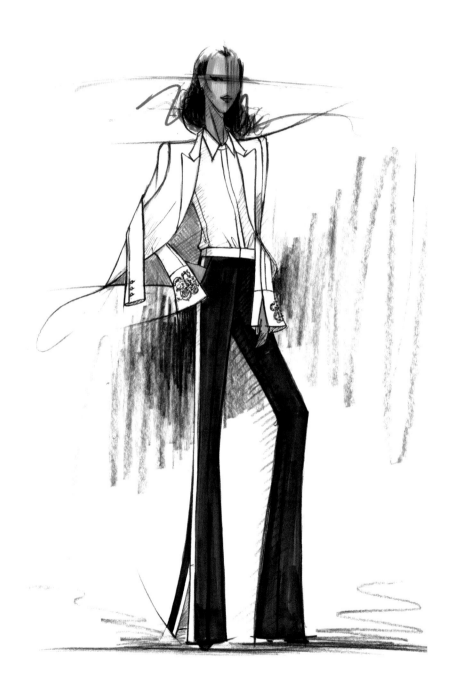

propriating men's clothing in an attempt to gain some semblance of equality, and the pieces weren't suited for our distinct shapes and curves. Women were finally able to don garments that evoked the same authority as men, but they still didn't look like they belonged in these newfound garments of prestige. Now, in place of its frumpy, mannish predecessor, the blazer of today is sexy and sophisticated. Spending a tiny bit more to have it tailored to fit your frame will prove to be a very wise investment. When a well-made, quality piece fits like a glove, you will find yourself wearing it in practically every aspect of your life, with everything from jeans and a tee to an embellished cocktail dress. A well-fitted blazer can be extremely forgiving and flattering, but not all blazers are created equal. Finding the most favorable fit starts when you purchase

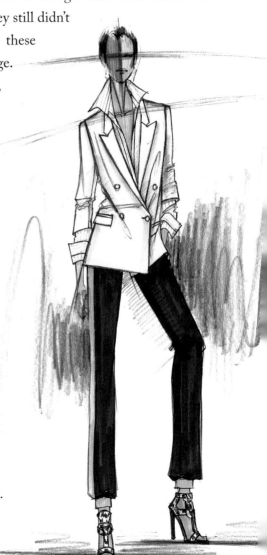

40

the piece at the store and ends when you pick it up from the tailor. When you're shopping for the perfect blazer, try on options in your regular top size, but always size up if the fit is slightly snug, because you can have it taken in but it's nearly impossible to let it out. For an optimal fit, visit a tailor you trust, and also ask them to adjust the hem to skim your low hips and take the sleeves out if they are too short. You should be able to button the blazer with ease, and be sure that the cross back fits your shoulders, is snug but not too tight, and does not extend past your actual shoulder. If it's a fitted blazer, there should also be a slight cinch at the waist to create the most flattering silhouette. Look for blazers with a high-cut armhole. At first you may think the garment does not fit or is too tight, but a high-cut armhole frames the body as slender, long, and as lean as possible. It gives the illusion of long, lean arms and a narrow back. Find shoulders that are sewn tight and are joined to the arm well, with either a small shoulder pad or rope inside to keep the shape for you. With the right fit, you'll end up looking and feeling like the smartest person in the room.

Many women think one blazer will work for every outfit, but there are so many different styles and types worth pairing with your regular wardrobe in dozens of different ways that it's worth stocking up.

THE TRENCH-STYLE DRESS

I designed a trench dress for a CFDA/*Vogue* program called "Runway to Green" that sold exclusively on Net-A-Porter. Each designer was asked to use only "green," environmentally safe materials in their creations, and I took the opportunity to design an Earth-friendly version of a piece I've always loved. I chose to design a trench-style A-line dress: a classic shape I've always believed to be the most universally flattering, accompanied by a patterned, large-swing skirt with the idea that it wears and travels well, especially in a blended fabric. Once the piece was designed and produced, Michelle Obama's stylist selected it to be worn by the First Lady.

I consider the trench dress to be a feminine equivalent to the men's suit. The idea behind the shape is that it is designed to promote function, comfort, and beauty, and it truly is flattering to all body shapes. I often use a solid trench dress as a blank palette to highlight whatever new accessory I have acquired, because the dress allows a jeweled heel or multicolored necklace to be the main focal point of the outfit and really become the spotlight, especially if the trench is not heavily designed. A few years back, I paired my own black silk trench dress with a jewel-toned turban and simple diamond-encrusted buckle heels and won a coveted spot on the *Vanity Fair* Best Dressed list for that simple yet strong accessory look.

The trench dress is formal enough to wear to the ballet or a cocktail party yet still casual enough to pair with flats and skinny jeans for a day at the office or out on the run. When I want to dress mine down a bit, I style it with a men's vintage brown leather belt, and the whole look instantly eases into something else altogether. When the waist is cinched tight, paired over a full-skirt trench, I adore how the shape creates the look of a femme fatale. Unless the extra fabric creates extra bulk, I always add pockets when designing trench dresses. Pockets add that desirable coolness and ease,

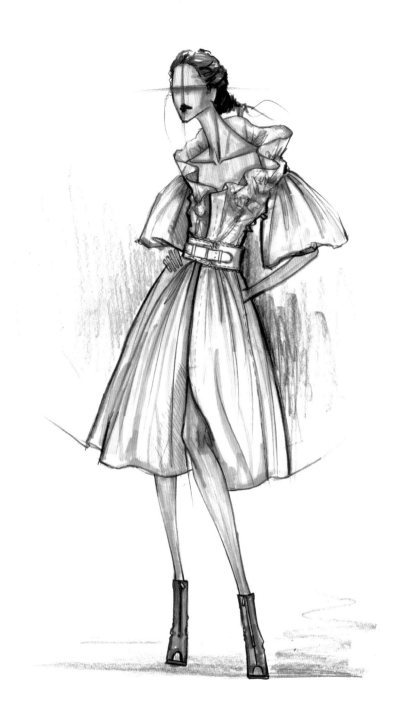

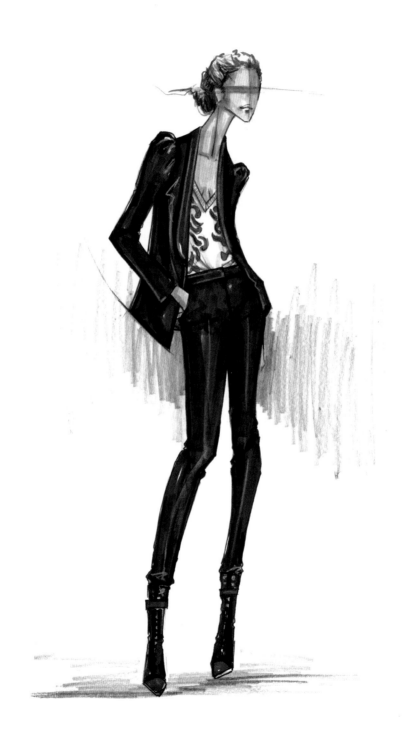

but they are also highly functional—they can hold a few key items without requiring the wearer to carry a purse, which is always much appreciated.

THE TAILORED TROUSERS

There is a notable difference between a pair of nice pants and a pair of custom-fit, tailored trousers, but the price points don't have to be worlds apart. For as little as twenty dollars, a skilled tailor can take in and let out an off-the-rack pair in all the right places. You'll look and, more important, you'll feel your best knowing that the material has been altered to hug you in the most flattering way possible. Trousers are extremely versatile, infusing a professional, sophisticated office look with just the right amount of cool, boyish style or the epitome of femininity when fit a bit more snug.

Various styles of trousers can flatter different body types; the key is how you alter them to your body.

45

Classic fem shape: Ensure the rise in the bum has the right scoop for your tush so it lifts and separates, giving the illusion of hours spent in the gym doing squats.

High-waisted: The higher the waist, the longer the leg. Ensure the waist is snug enough to hold in the tummy and create a long, lean-looking wall of a torso—the illusion works wonders, especially with heavier fabric. For short-

Tip: Look for traditional menswear silhouettes, in men's styles, which can many times be less expensive than women's clothing; then tailor them to fit your curves perfectly.

legged girls, taper the ankle and show a bit of skin so the fabric does not overwhelm.

Wide-leg: Ensure the fabric hangs straight down from the widest part of your body—usually your low hip. This will give the illusion of long, lean legs. Also allow the waistline to skim your hips, similar to a boyfriend jean; a tight waistline with wide leg pants will add weight. I reserve that shape for the skinniest version of myself only.

Tapered: Good on everyone—add invisible ankle zippers on the inside or outside of the ankle for easy access in and out and to ensure a snug ankle fit.

Cropped: Good on everyone. Mid-calf is the goal. Super easy when you envision Audrey Hepburn and simply channel her, replacing a twin set with your own signature top.

THE RIGHT ACCESSORIES

I have a tendency to dress very feminine; it is quite easy for me to go there quickly and without even realizing it. What I've realized, however, is that I feel off balance when I'm dressed in a completely feminine style head to toe. Although I greatly admire feminine flourishes and embellished folds and pleats, unless I am balancing them with something opposite in nature, I don't feel like myself. I either add more masculine accessories to an otherwise softer look 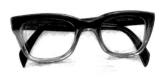 to even things up a bit or take off some of the overtly feminine touches. When looking for a hint of masculinity, I seek out an equilibrium I can only get through my menswear pieces: oversized watch, loafers, oxford shoes, or a handsome carryall. I love eyeglasses, too; depending on your style, they can completely transform your look. I wear them in a way that's anything but dainty, opting for frames that are bold and strong, and remind me a bit of a 1950s professor. The right accessories can create that necessary harmony between sharp and soft, edgy and classic, whether you're headed to the office or out for leisure.

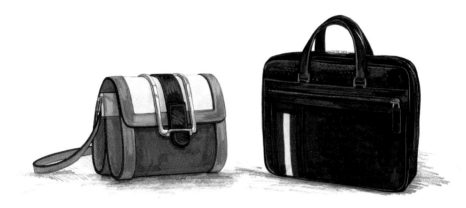

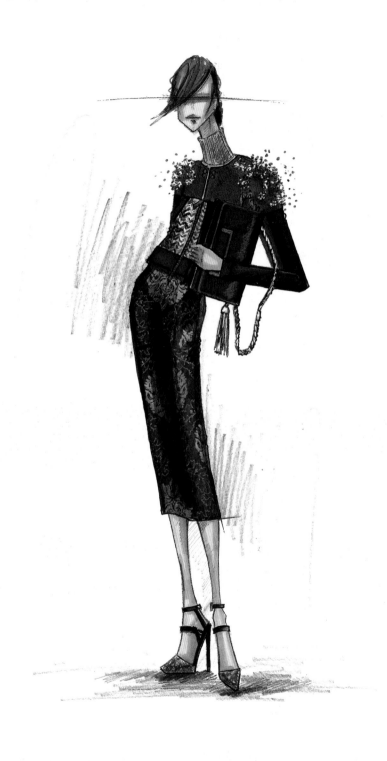

· 3 ·

THE ART OF MIXING PATTERNS AND STYLES

I want everyone to wear what they want and mix it in their own way. That, to me, is what is modern.

—KARL LAGERFELD

Being the daughter of a statuesque Dutch mother and an Indian immigrant father covered in tattoos taught me how to blend, mix, and integrate influences and styles like no design class ever could. I always felt a deep sense of attachment to both sides of my family and a profound identification with both cultures. Wearing influences from both sides of my genetic landscape always seemed to be the most natural way for me to celebrate my mixed heritage and pay homage to both my Dutch and my Indian roots.

I quickly found that seemingly contradictory staples from both of my cultures actually complemented each other in an incredibly interesting way. I found ways to incorporate my tan leather Indian-inspired sandals with long, traditional peasant skirts I'd seen in photos of locals in the Netherlands. It was eye-opening and inspiring to realize how much beauty can be found in atypical pairings, and the eclectic combinations not only connected me even closer to my biracial identity, but were more interesting than the likely pairings I could have opted for. Today in my designs, I mix prints that complement one another, which I feel adds life, depth, and vibrancy to an outfit. When done right, blending is extremely flattering, and any fear of clashing is quickly quelled by the sight of how certain prints and shapes actually accentuate just the right curves and camouflage the rest. The trick to brilliant blending is, as with everything in life, to always incorporate balance. When going bold with a crisp graphic style, even out the overall look with something delicate or ladylike, such as a floral or washed out tie-dye. Do not underestimate the importance of color and tone: the easiest way to mix and match is to settle on a hue that works with your skin tone and plays up your best features. For example, play up eye color, go for a complementary tone; same for your hair and complexion: Beautiful mocha complexion? Try a shot of cobalt to complement your skin tone. Once you have your color palette down, which really requires holding things up to you in a mirror and being honest about what highlights and what does not, select pieces in varying shades of that hue to create a more current, layered look. If you have a hard time stepping out of your neutral-tones-only comfort zone, and the idea of blending prints and patterns seems overwhelming, start small with a floral shoe or patterned purse. Just a little pop of pattern goes a long way, and once you feel comfortable flaunting a bit of personality, you may be emboldened to go bigger and brighter.

When you are ready to mix your prints or stripes, I have a few rules I let loosely guide me:

Balance a graphic with something lighter in feel. A graphic could be anything with direct harsh lines or shapes, from grid stripes to

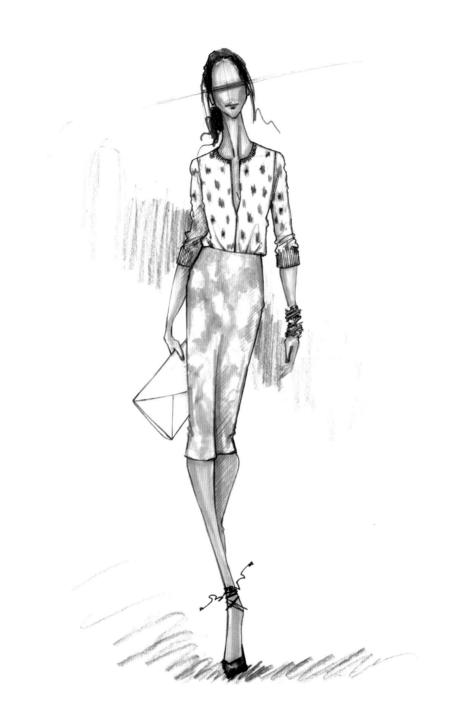

polka dots. Lighter-feeling prints are just that: washed-out animal prints or painterly florals. If you want to mix like prints together, such as stripes with stripes, choose similar-colored pieces and mix the width and size of the stripes. Same for mixing similar prints together in one look, like florals; choose colors that go well together and just mix the scale of the actual flowers in the print. Once you feel confident in those choices you can move on to more risk-taking print combinations.

THE CREATION

Mixing, blending, and reworking aren't only applied to material things. As women, it's often our natural inclination to care for everyone around us and neglect our own well-being. The older we grow and the more we evolve, the bigger our circle of loved ones becomes, and the less time we have to focus on our own self-care. Placing ourselves so far down the priority list is neither a smart nor a healthy strategy—not for ourselves, and not for those we love. I like to look at the juggle of life as an opportunity to cohesively blend all the aspects of my life, making sure one area supports or complements the other. The trick, I believe, is building that base from within you.

Oprah Winfrey once said that when she puts herself first, she can take care of others best. I fully agree and have observed the evidence in my personal life over and over again. The truth in her statement deeply resonates with me, and ever since coming across the quote I constantly remind myself of this sentiment and make conscious efforts to ensure my needs are being met, even on the most basic level. As a working mother, friend, daughter, and partner, I know those words are easier said than done. But just like everything else worth accomplishing, mastering good self-care involves practice, repetition, and dedication. When I first started applying this idea seriously, I had to schedule my self-care into my day. Whether it was a workout, a bath, a massage, or even just fifteen minutes alone in a room to breathe and re-center, I blocked out a portion of my busy day and focused on strengthening me. It was difficult to stick to at first, and even felt a little selfish. I soon started to reap the benefits, and so did everyone I cared for. Being better rested, more relaxed, and rejuvenated, I was less distracted by my problems, and could give my all to those who really needed me.

As a designer, I always consider it a goal and priority of mine to create clothes for women who, like me, are performing in the ultimate juggling act called life. Through my designs, I strive to make the dream of looking and acting like we have it all together slightly more within reach by producing pieces that are sophisticated and uncomplicated. We need nothing that further complicates our lives, particularly in our wardrobe. I am a firm believer that getting dressed should be enjoyable—putting together the perfect outfit should feel like another moment of self-care, not another chore to drain your energy and suck needed minutes from your day. I want women to look forward to putting themselves together, feel beautiful and confident in the pieces they choose, and go out into the world presenting the most poised, polished versions of themselves possible—which I believe leads to their best work possible.

Blending plays a huge part in the fun factor of getting dressed. A fail-proof tip to look strong, savvy, and fashion-forward is to mix and match hues and textures. When I see a woman who is able to blend various patterns in a way that is visually appealing and works for her body, I see a woman who can keep it all together and make things work in ways that reach beyond fashion. It's safe to stick to neutrals, but it's rarely noteworthy unless paired with something boisterous in feel, even if it is just a handbag or shoes. One of the most important parts of putting together an outfit is to do it in a way that is unique to your individual tastes, traits, and character. I want every woman to feel comfortable and confident putting herself out into the world and voicing her beliefs, fighting for what she wants, and doing it with self-respect. A woman who is willing to do that should also be game to step outside the box with her fashion choices, and play with the patterns and colors she connects to. Clothing choices are often dismissed as a superficial detail, but they're an important signifier of your self-esteem and willingness to show the world what you're made of.

On the surface, we as women have many layers and labels, wearing a million different hats and fulfilling an unbelievable array of roles. As we move about our everyday lives, it's easy to pigeonhole those around us and categorize them based on the most surface-level traits: she's a mother; that woman's a waitress; this lady is a teacher. But there is so much more than meets the eye when it comes to people, and to women specifically. We embody so many traits and emotions, and take on so many responsibilities that go under the radar, that our inner spirit is often obscured by the most obvious roles we fulfill and our outermost layers. When it comes to style, I appreciate quirky little touches that tell the observer, "This is who my spirit is. I'm not one-dimensional. I'm more than a predictable pantsuit." The challenge is always to create a look that appears pulled together while showcasing an engaging personality. With this in mind, I sought to design a versatile time-saver for women who, like me, have way too much to accomplish in a single day, but are committed to completing it all. I wanted to design something that looked well thought-out and strategically planned, but in truth was as easy as zipping into one piece before heading out the door. My goal was to provide an alternative to wearing a plain, run-of-the-mill office dress or anything else that others could consider "basic" (which has apparently become the most dreaded of descriptors). With all those goals in mind, I designed what I think is the ideal foundation for the ultimate expressive, yet professional and polished any-day-of-the-week go-to ensemble. I ended up starting with the elements of a tasteful, staple skirt suit and mixing two graphic prints in one garment.

The end result became a personal favorite that has been included in every collection for the last ten years: the mixed-print dress. One of my first mixed-print dresses had a pencil-style skirt constructed from black-and-white tweed, providing tactile richness. The top featured a washed-out navy and oxblood print with black polka dots. The circles in the top shell blended smoothly against the small squares in the tweed. An oxblood tuxedo-inspired cummerbund grounded the two prints, and the finished garment reflected a unique look and feel I had not designed before. This being one piece makes blending a no-brainer, because the work has already

57

been done for the woman wearing it. With this dress, there is one less decision to be made or color to be considered when it comes to getting ready to take on the world. In fact, the zipper was purposely sewn onto the outside of the garment to make it easier for a woman to get in and out of it herself without having to ask a partner or child to zip it up for her. I tried to consider every last detail of design in order to make this the most functional, freeing, descriptive garment in a woman's closet.

THE INSPIRATION

One of the most thrilling calls of my career came unexpectedly at six o'clock in the morning. On the other end of the line was one of my marketing team members, speaking a mile a minute, and excitedly relaying details of who had worn our mixed-print dress that was out at the time. Someone from my office had come across a photo of First Lady Michelle Obama giving a speech in San Francisco while wearing our signature mixed-print shift dress—the one I'd created with the intention of enabling all women to run their world a bit more effortlessly. Mixed emotions raced through my head as I was over the moon and grateful, as well as proud of my team. Realizing that one of the most scrutinized women in our country felt comfortable and confident in my dress made me feel more than proud—it completely bolstered my own self-confidence and inspired me to continue on this path. That FLOTUS is also so closely watched in the world at large and chose to wear this particular design made me feel accomplished, validated, and fully realized.

The milestone moment was also an incredible confirmation that what I was setting out to do with my designs was being achieved. It can be difficult to see the big picture and the end result when you're so hyper-focused on the minute details of a particular project. You know that *you* think it's a good idea with endless potential, but when you put it out in the world it can be viewed in a different way. Even the best intentions executed improperly can wind up as fails. Seeing my design come to life in such a spectacular way was encouraging and rejuvenating, giving me more inspiration and drive to continue doing what I love— helping women get dressed simply and easily and get on with the things that matter in life.

The type of woman I design for wears many hats and takes many chances, allowing her ideas to direct her journey. That multifaceted nature is reflected in her wardrobe: she's not just wearing one look, in one color, with one fabric. Through our fashion choices, we can let the world know there is much more to us than what is on the surface. We all get labeled as we move through the world. We become associated with our roles and our depth is often stripped away, so that we're moving through the world as caricatures of our true, complicated, interesting, individual selves. My goal with my designs is to grant women the opportunity to break free of the oppressive molds we often find ourselves in, and chicly, elegantly, uniquely represent our true selves in all our multilayered, complex beauty. I want women to signal to the world that they are more than their jobs, their families, their bank accounts—they are intelligent, sensual, soft, contradictory, and magnetic rare spirits. When I saw the First Lady, the woman who inspires the women whom I design for, wearing my dress, I immediately knew that particular goal had been met.

60

THE PHILOSOPHY

While I want my clothes to hint at who I am from the inside out, at the same time, I don't want them to overpower me. Clothes are meant to be an extension of who we are, but they shouldn't upstage us. They shouldn't stand out before we do. I have a hard time with this occasionally, because finding clothes that are fitted and flattering and play up my best features can be a challenge. I would design them for myself but lack of time prevents me from using my atelier as a private tailor shop. Being five feet ten and large busted means I am constantly aware of my size and the length of my hemline. Certain tops (yes, you, halters) just don't look the same on a woman with an A-cup versus someone with a D-cup. As much as I respect a miniskirt on other people, it can quickly make me appear to be reaching for the look of a genre or age that I'm not actually trying to achieve. A short skirt and platforms look quite different on someone who is a petite five feet two than they do on me. Because of that fact, I abide by one major rule when considering eye-catching patterns, prints, shapes, and styles: if my outfit walks into a room before I do, that's a negative.

Our physical attributes should always be considered, but they shouldn't be roadblocks, either. There are just certain workarounds that all women should be aware of when trying to incorporate a trend or look that may not be as intuitive a fit for her body compared with others. Being tall doesn't mean I can't wear a mini. With an opaque tight and an androgynous top to balance me, I can grab attention by what I'm saying—not what others are distracted by, whether it's my outfit or my body. The simplest way I break down the art of blending to women is to apply the same logic that is fundamental to makeup application in order to prevent us from donning a full-on over-contoured clown face: play up one particular part, and keep the rest understated and simple. Going for a dark, smoky eye? Keep the lips light. Opting for a bold cherry-red shade on the lips? Perhaps try a lighter eye with mascara only. The same rules apply to style: if you're showing off your legs, keep it covered on top, and vice versa. Too much is simply that.

———

THIS PLUS THAT:
Blending Tips & Tricks

Remember my tips for mixing prints—try mixing opposite feelings like florals with stripes or animal prints with graphics. If you want to wear stripes only, try mixing different width stripes within the same color family. It is all about balance, as is everything in life.

ILLUSIONS: LONGER LEGS, WAIST, TORSO

Color blocking is a wonderful way to attract the eye, accentuate a feature, or create an illusion. I like using a bold color to cinch the waist on a boxy style or to ground a busy look. By adding a bright collar to a quiet blouse or an eye-popping saturation to an off-the-shoulder shirt, you can draw attention to your décolletage or shoulders and away from an area you do not want highlighted.

Blending isn't just about prints and tones: you can combine styles and trends, too. If you're a very feminine girl, balance that style with something edgy like a studded pair of earrings or clutch.

What it means to mix high and low—fashion is hardly ever modern unless you mix it.

Aim to blend tones, not exact colors.

Mix gold with silver. It shows confidence and displays modernity.

A must-have item for mixing is a nude shoe. A skin-tone pump will elongate your line, making you look as tall as possible while creating a balance for busy prints and textures.

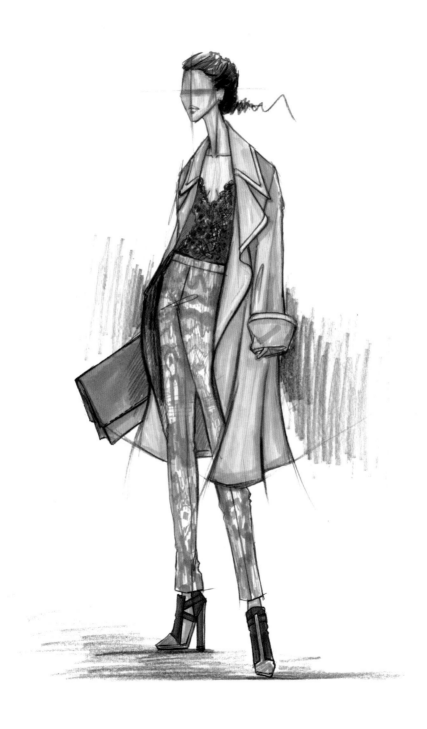

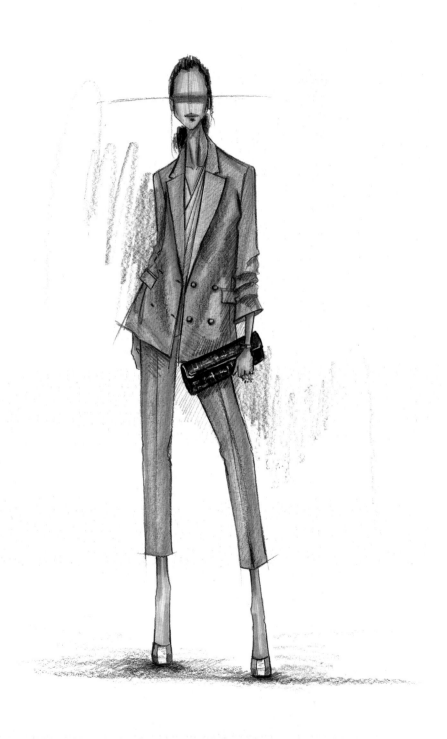

· 4 ·

INVESTING
WISELY
IN YOUR
WARDROBE

Always keep your eyes open. Keep watching. Because whatever you can see can inspire you.

—GRACE CODDINGTON,
CREATIVE DIRECTOR AT *VOGUE*

Saving for and investing in timeless, well-made accessories is an educated move your wallet will appreciate and creates luxurious looks everyone will appreciate. However, there's nothing wrong with buying whimsical, vibrant costume jewelry to elevate an outfit and add your individual fingerprint to your look.

In the industry there is a term for inexpensive, lower-quality items: "fast fashion." Purchasing clothes or accessories made to sell with this intent does have its perks. There are times when it just makes more sense to save the splurge and go lower-cost. For example, it's an incredibly wise choice to opt for an affordable version of a trend you're on the fence about. Intrigued by that designer neon chartreuse purse or those floral print jeans that retail for the equivalent of a car payment? It might make more sense to buy affordable versions first to test-drive the trends and see how you feel about them after a few wears. There's nothing worse than investing in an of-the-moment piece, only to find the moment is far more fleeting than you'd hoped—no sense in mourning the loss of your much needed $. When it comes to staple pieces that you know suit you well and perfectly complement your shape, or items that you know you want to hang on to for many years to come, the fact is that you're going to save money over the long run by spending a little on fast fashion to test trends, and then buying quality pieces when you are certain that you can afford it!

One thing I like to consider when determining the worthiness of an item is its cost-per-wear. Knowing this number is an excellent way to simultaneously keep an eye on your bank account and reevaluate your closet. Here's how it works: the next time you're contemplating a high-priced fashion investment, estimate how many times you'll wear the item in one month. Multiply it by twelve to figure out how often you'll wear it in the next year. Multiply that number by the amount of years you anticipate keeping the item. Still with me? Now divide the cost on the price tag by that magic number and you'll have an estimated cost-per-wear. There are no right or wrong answers when it comes to cost-per-wear, and your opinion on what constitutes a valuable, wear-all-the-time item is of course subjective. You have to decide for yourself ahead of time what makes sense for your budget, your lifestyle, and your wardrobe. If you're in lust with a perfectly tailored pantsuit but your day-to-day doesn't typically call for such a corporate uniform, you may want to reconsider and put your money where you'll get the most long-term bang for your buck. Spend most days typing away on your laptop in the neighborhood café? Then investing in a gorgeous leather laptop bag and a classic pair of ballet flats may make more sense. It all comes down to

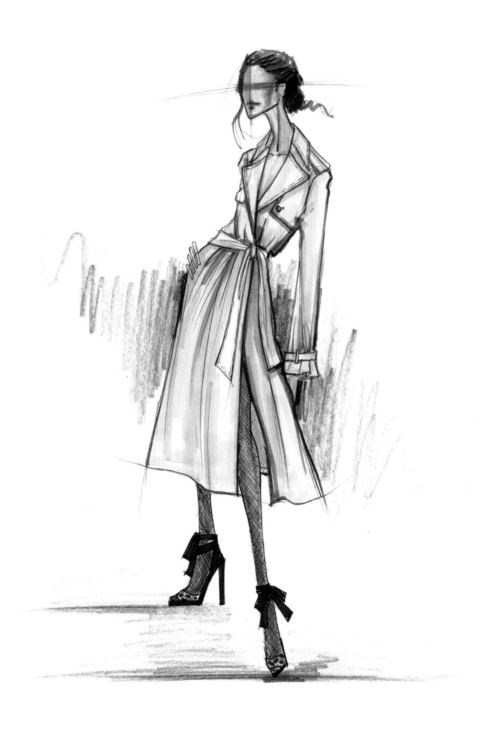

your individual style and where you're willing to invest. In my case, well-made designer shoes are where I want lasting quality and head-turning style. And while it's never easy to lay down the credit card when faced with a higher-than-your-average-shoe price tag, it just so happens one of my very oldest pairs is still in rotation, coming out to about five cents per wear! That type of math is brilliantly simple in thought: quality x's style equals savings. And I am absolutely just as in love with them as I was the day I laid eyes on them.

THE CREATION

The moment I saw them, I knew. They were the ones: my very first pair of Manolo Blahniks. While most girls my age during those college years might have opted for a flashy platform, I chose the single-sole heel because it was a classic option, a style that I knew had stood the test of time and would continue to endure as a time-less staple. I had a bit of a Carrie Bradshaw moment the second I examined them up close, admiring their structure. Once I slipped them on, I instantly felt both cultured and at ease—always a good sign when considering a new addition to your life. Eyeing them in the mirror, I envisioned them taking me to interviews, dinner dates, parties, and an endless series of events over years to come. The frame was strong and sturdy, and that solid foundation seemed to strengthen my stance as well, as I stood there, evaluating the pur-chase. I somehow felt more competent and commanding, but still sexy and ultra-feminine. Adding to the versatility of the shape, the chocolate brown hue was dark enough to pass for black, increasing the wearability potential exponentially. That they were pony hair gave the shoes a bit of edge, allowing them to stand out in a sea of leather and suede.

This was no frivolous impulse purchase. In fact, I had been planning it and thinking it out months in advance. Between running to class and cramming for tests, I worked as the assistant manager at a store in the local mall, saving up every penny I could, after using the majority of my paycheck for rent, bills, and other essentials. After months of penny-pinching, the dream shoes were actually within my reach without putting myself at risk for bankruptcy: they were on the shelf at Neiman Marcus's annual last-call sale, where designer items were priced at up to 70 percent off. I somehow instinctively had the sense to know that investing in one pair of beautifully made Manolos a year would serve me better in the long run than buying multiple pairs of inexpensive knockoff shoes that would come and go and potentially cause a slew of painful blisters along the way. I came to know this through experience, trial and error. Over the years I had tried every which way to make the cheap shoes I could afford work, but they never lasted and they hurt—both my pride and my feet. So my dedicated planning paid off. I still wear those very shoes to this day, and I feel worldly, wise, and classic every time I slip them on. In fact, I wore them to my very first meeting with Anna Wintour.

THE INSPIRATION

Aside from the common "hello"s and "how are you"s of everyday small talk, people in the fashion industry have a particular way of getting to know each other: we share our first "Anna" moment. Anna Wintour is, after all, the most powerful person in fashion. "What was your first Anna moment?" It's incredibly telling to know what a fellow industry insider's first interaction with Anna Wintour was like. For decades, Ms. Wintour has stood at the helm of *Vogue* and transformed the way we think about fashion. Meeting her for the first time is a true milestone, and a memorable one. Early in my career as a designer, when André Leon Talley, former editor-at-large at *Vogue,* visited me in one of my first showrooms to view my collection, he decided right away I needed to present it to the head of *Vogue* herself. I was honored and more than a little nervous. This opportunity of a lifetime came with one major catch: I'd have to present my 2006 fall collection to her in less than three days. My anxiety, of course, was at an all-time high, as I quickly prepared for the meeting. In some cases less time to prepare is for the best; it forces you to get it done and the self-doubt has to be pushed to the side to get the work completed.

My nerves were unbearable as I wheeled a rolling rack of my designs down crowded New York City streets to the Condé Nast building and up the service elevator, waited in the lobby, and then eventually maneuvered into a narrow corridor to meet with Ms. Wintour.

I couldn't afford a top model to showcase my collection then; however, the agency sent me several of their best girls to don my designs because the chance to get in front of Anna was an epic opportunity for everyone. In fact, everyone who helped prepare for my Anna moment worked for free, just for the chance to get close to the legendary editor in chief and because that is what you do when opportunity comes: you work toward it and through it with all of the help you can. Plus, that is how respected she is; everyone in her field wants to learn from her and work with her.

As I was scrambling to appear professional in the presence of a legend, the hallways were so narrow that one could only walk in front of or behind a rolling rack. My team and I were blocking foot traffic, so my design assistant and models waited with me in a tiny (and incredibly well-stocked) sample closet until it was time to present.

I wore my own design that day: the trench dress I described earlier, featuring leather laser cutouts on the skirt—a design that has proved its worth to me time and time again. To complement the dress, I chose to wear the pony hair Manolos I'd saved so long for as a student. It was a way of speaking to my younger self and saying, "We are at *Vogue*! I'm so proud of you!"

While waiting in the closet, I remember my assistant asking, "Are you okay? How are you feeling?" She most definitely could see on my face that I was a complete mess, unsure whether to pass out, cry, or run from the claustrophobic space altogether. I knew then I had to snap out of my stupor and pull it together. I reminded myself this was a fight-or-flight moment. I was determined to fight for my self-respect after spending so long working for others—the decade-plus I had put in working in retail and the seven years that followed helping to create a clothing company for my previous employers. Working for oneself, making the decisions and directing the entire brand, is such a risk yet such a rewarding journey, and the journey had led me to the office of one of my idols.

We were summoned into Anna's office, and down the narrow halls we walked. Her desk was front and center, its back to the windows. I scanned the perimeter of the room for editors I knew. André was there, a familiar face that helped ease a fraction of my anxiety. Everyone was all business, eager to see my presentation and get on with the show. No small talk, no time to kill, just me and my designs, and my chance to show my work and my dedication to what I believed in. I stood at the center of the room and knew I did not have much time to get my story across. I didn't have a lot of time to describe my motivation or to demonstrate my authentic, deep-rooted obsession with all things fashion, and the lack of expository information made me even more nervous because I desperately wanted her to know how passionate I was. I went right into speaking about the clothes, which the girls quickly changed into and out of after modeling each piece. As soon as I started talking about the clothes, my nerves subsided. I was speaking about the one thing I truly had no doubt about—my passion: the fashion business. My earnestness and confidence were coming through loud and clear, and I could feel it because it was authentic and straight from the heart. A few pieces in, Anna asked me what stores I was in, which ones I wanted to be in, and what my future business plans looked like. I knew that the only reason she would ask these questions was because she recognized my potential, thought I was viable, and perhaps even sensed I could create a solid, successful business. This awareness had a strong influence on me but at the time I did my best to conceal it by remaining composed. Ms. Wintour went on to pepper me with a few more business-related questions and then asked what I'd be wearing to the annual Met Ball, the Oscars of the fashion industry. It was 2006 and it would be my second time attending. She encouraged me not to wear black, so I wore cream, with bright orange custom Manolos—my good-luck shoe designer.

The only way I knew the meeting was officially over was when one of the editors stepped forward to ask, "Can I help you get your samples together?" My fifteen minutes were up. As we were leaving the offices of *Vogue,* an editor friend of mine whispered "great job" in my ear, and the compliment gave me a sense of ambition and a reason to live up to the standard that I had established. It showed me how to take the lead in a way I had not realized before. In understanding this I discovered how important it would be for me to do this for others as well. The kindness in that moment had a lasting influence, instilling leadership within me. Later, André would tell me he was honored to be the one who recommended I see Anna and that he was impressed by how well-spoken and prepared I came across. André doesn't mince words and speaks the truth whether he's upset or happy, confirming I was in a solid place.

My first Anna moment far surpassed my expectations. Just being lucky enough to have this type of experience surpassed any early expectations I had about my career, but holding my own and presenting the best version of myself was among one of the most memorable milestones early in my career. She was extremely supportive that day, and over the years to come she became someone I called on regularly for advice and guidance. As my mentor, she has given me priceless wisdom on my career, and as a successful, strong, brilliant woman, she's served as a true inspiration.

Anxiously anticipating my presentation with Ms. Wintour that day, in the *Vogue* sample closet, I could have never imagined that the design I wore, which evoked so much strength from within me, would give the same empowered energy to Oprah Winfrey herself—she would later wear the same dress on her "Best of Oscar" wrap-up show.

THE PHILOSOPHY

Those Manolos I bought so many years earlier served me well both in moments that I wanted to remember forever and in times I'd sooner forget. No matter where I was in my life, they were a consistent staple I could depend on to match almost any combination of clothing; make me look sharp, professional, poised, and put together; and, above all, feel completely at ease in my own skin and empowered enough to radiate that inner spirit out to the world. (Yes, shoes can empower!) That experience solidified the fact that I don't feel good buying anything for my body that doesn't make me feel proud of that item and of myself while wearing it. For while designer labels and perfectly tailored pieces look exquisite on the outside, their real value is in their ability to evoke the wearer's sense of self-worth and spirit. Confidence makes everyone look and feel savvy, powerful, and alluring beyond words.

THE ORDER OF INVESTING

Quality trumps quantity in every circumstance, especially when it comes to staple accessories. When it comes to investing, I will suggest to my daughters that they invest in the same order I did, starting with shoes and in time moving on to handbags and, later, to a watch.

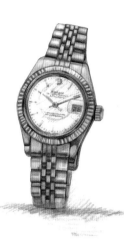

SHOES

One of the most helpful hints of shopping advice I have, whether you're on a budget or not, is to get to know the salespeople in your favorite department stores. Building and fostering these close relationships is in the best interest of both sides; while you will receive early notice of sales, have a last item in your size put on hold, or be notified the moment an exact style you've been in search of hits the floor, the salespeople are accomplishing their goal of making a sale, and moving closer to hitting the numbers assigned to them by their managers. In contrast, by shopping in designers' individual boutiques and shops, you can often ask salespeople to order custom pieces for you that you wouldn't be able to order on your own or even through a larger store. Either way, having connections in retail shops has definite perks, not to mention that these hardworking fellow style-savvy insiders are some of the coolest, kindest people you'll meet in the fashion world. Sales associates know exactly when their departments will be having a major blowout sale, and they'll happily tip you off to VIP events if you're a loyal customer. They also

77

know when things will be 20 percent off versus 50 percent off, and they can save you the exasperation of impulsively grabbing an item on sale, only to find it retailing for half the price later on. There is nothing more frustrating than returning to a store weeks later to find the product you purchased further reduced from what you paid, and beating yourself up for assuming you'd gotten an amazing deal. Buddy up with your favorite salesperson, and he or she will hook you up with insider knowledge that will spare your sanity and your paycheck.

So how do you find the person in the department who just *gets* you? Getting to know the right salesperson means finding someone who understands your style, has enough fashion experience to know what will complement your figure, shape, and lifestyle, and can be brutally honest when necessary, even if it means losing out on a potential big-ticket sale. They should be able to identify your tastes after a few heart-to-heart shopping sessions and understand what works for your body. A stellar salesperson keeps track of his or her client's sizes and knows to jot down important dates, such as their birthday or anniversary. Last year, I was searching for a pair of sand-colored snakeskin pumps with a sexy pointed toe and a single sole. I looked everywhere but I just could not track down an ideal pair; there are great expectations placed on my uniform staples! Often the simplest pieces are the hardest to find. It was a sales associate at Saks who really understood me and knew what to put aside. She knew what I was searching for and called me the moment they came in. I was—and still am—very appreciative of her helpful and kind customer service skills.

HANDBAGS

When I was pregnant with my second daughter and at the stage where my body was getting very uncomfortable, I was also working full-time and just a few years into starting my own company, feeling overwhelmed with to-do lists and managing all that I had to get done in the day. Suffice it to say, I wasn't at my very best. That is, until I was surprised by a true Cinderella moment courtesy of André Leon Talley. André was sent out—as a favor—to scour the city for the most beautiful bags to shower me with much-needed and -appreciated feel-glam gifts. With each tote, clutch, and saddle came a handwritten note detailing what kind of outfits the purse would best complement and for which oc-

> *Three styles of handbags worth saving for:*
>
> EVERYDAY
> CARRYALL
>
> DAY-TO-NIGHT
> SHOULDER BAG
>
> UPSCALE
> CLUTCH

casions. It was the most thoughtful sentiment I'd ever received, and it of course instantly shifted my outlook, boosted my self-esteem, and reminded me that feeling super chic has nothing to do with squeezing into a sample size. Luckily, André has even more tips to help sort out our quest for the perfect handbag, check them out on pages 82-83.

WATCH

While our first inclination is always to consider our tastes, it's important also to think about lifestyle when it comes to buying a watch. What is your purpose for owning one? Is it for functionality or for flash factor? Would you consider yourself conservative or sporty? Is your style vintage or modern, more masculine or feminine? All these questions are ones to answer for yourself before you start seeking out the perfect complement to your wrist.

A watch is a very personal thing, after all—it combines the functionality of an accessory with the beauty of fine jewelry, and there's a lot to consider when you're in the market for one you'll want to keep in mint condition for years to come. Not only will you wear it for a lifetime, but it could also be passed down to your children, maybe even your children's children. With that said, the timepiece you choose should be timeless and represent what you stand for. I have wanted the classic rectangle-face Cartier watch for as long as I can remember, spotting it on a rather intelligent and style-savvy individual years ago. When friends of mine were gifted watches or bought them for themselves, I would imagine which one I would choose—could I afford what I wanted? A brown alligator strap, rectangular faced, clean, simple, and elegant classic Cartier. The shape worn by Louis Cartier himself, the Tank. Seeing both sophisticated men and women wearing them, the watches symbolized strength, beauty, and history. I knew it was the design for me well before I wore it. I wanted this watch not only because it literally goes with everything from jeans to cocktail attire but also for what it stands for. Before I was making my own money, there was no way for me to have the opportunity to treat myself to this accessory. It wasn't until after all the hard work paid off that I was able to call the watch mine. It felt incredible to work toward something I'd admired for so long and actually be able to buy it for myself. Along with the thrill of designing pieces I know other women will be proud to purchase and have for many years, it too is an extraordinary and gratifying feeling that never gets old, to care for yourself and gift yourself every now and then.

When struggling with the decision of a pricey purchase, I consider the 3 "Well"s:

WELL MADE: Are the materials high quality? Will it pass the test of time with numerous wears and washes?

WELL EXECUTED: Is the stitching straight and well sewn? Is the hardware sewn correctly?

WELL FITTING: Do the cut and fabric do my body any favors, or is it not right for my shape?

If one of the "Well"s does not check off, my credit card stays in my wallet. Each and every time I hold myself to that standard I am happy with the decision I made to hold back. Especially when the credit card statement comes!

Handbags 101 BY ANDRÉ LEON TALLEY

The **braided clutch** owes a debt to the classic invented by the famous leather house of Bottega Veneta. This woven leather clutch is ideal for dressing up any wardrobe look, including a pair of jeans, with flats and a great jacket or top. It's also meant for all seasons, and goes anywhere from a wedding to a casual date. Not for boardroom appointments. Then again, if you own the company, you can carry it around the clock for your cellphone, keys, and lipstick.

A **tricolor roomy clutch** with metal ornamentation is a perfect all-purpose clutch, from 9 a.m. to 9 p.m. and later. This bag packed in one's suitcase can go with everything, every moment of one's business as well as quality downtime day. For an interview, for a job, for lunch, dinner, or cocktails, if kept in perfect condition, it's a great investment and empowers a look with authority.

The **boho sack** is as casual as casual gets. Ideal for travel and just daily junkets: great for relaxed weekend choices and holiday travel, it's great even with a full pleated dress and no sleeves. It holds everything one could possibly need. It expresses the best kind of handbag from town to country.

The **double-handled saddlebag** with silver metal details is an appropriate bag for every day, from morning school runs to the office, to afternoon chores, to a visit to the spa or yoga. It's a great bag to pair with a pantsuit for lunch. Also elegant on the shoulder for travel. What is wonderful about the shape is that it converts easily from a functional, work-executive handbag to weekend brunch and errand casual.

The elegant **framed pocketbook**: one could find in its evolution from the forties throughout the fifties, and its sudden return in the new century, a bag that demands respect. It's for formal dressing, yet it can look great with a skirt, sweater, accessorized,

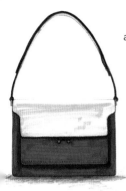

and with heels of any height. It's perfect for the dressiest of coats, suits, or day dresses as well as dinner. While not something you would select for effortless weekend dressing, unless it's a simple silhouette in a dress, or separates, it's got a Princess Grace vibe without being too elegant. It's serious but shouldn't be taken that seriously. Great inside a large tote if required for a midday lunch.

An **executive documents tote** with outer zipper compartments is double-handled and an accessory that escorts well any elegant shoulder bag for work-related duties. It's not a bag that acts on its own. Elegant for official papers and looks great as a woman's executive brief bag. It's perfect for all official appointments.

Of course, you wouldn't show up for dinner with that bag.

A **soft duffle bag**, the most ideal easy office-to-gym-to-travel bag. It can be dressed up or down: with a dressy coat for lunch, with jeans for travel—it's all-purpose, all seasons.

The **tote**: another way to organize briefs or official documents, carry a small swagger of a quilted Chanel bag inside, carry makeup bags, and just the best bag shape ever for a woman who lives with her life beside her, neatly housed in a sleek tote instead of a weekend canvas toile bucket tote. You always look sleek with a handbag that has this much room and style.

The **quilted chain bag is always** Chanel and should always be an authentic Chanel. Mademoiselle invented the style and it's an investment wardrobe must.

Women have wardrobes in colors and sizes, yet a basic black or white can meet every possible need in a woman's life. It's roomy, neat, and has inside compartments that help a woman stay organized.

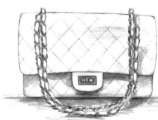

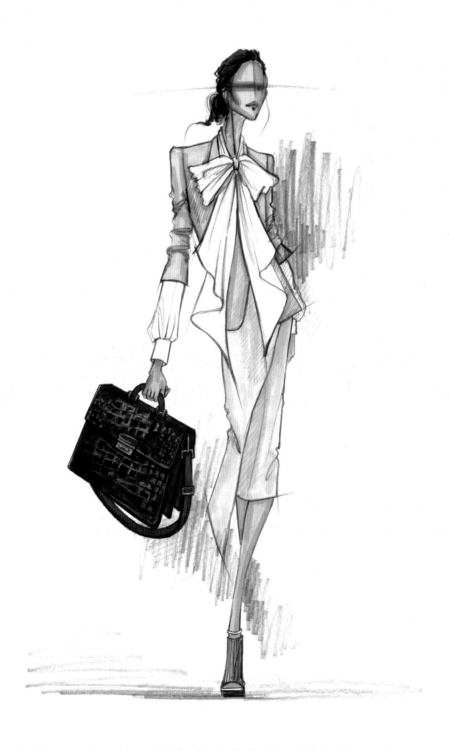

· 5 ·

DRESSING UP

CONVEYING STRENGTH
THROUGH STYLE

*If you can't
be better than
your competition,
just dress better.*

—ANNA WINTOUR

W hen I first arrived in New York City, I immediately took notice of the way New York women carried themselves—it was impossible not to.

It seemed like almost everyone had an elevated sense of self-knowledge combined with a uniqueness, regardless of whether they were actual CFOs or Coffee Fetchers Only. The self-assuredness was palpable and inspirational. Those women I observed when I first moved to the city encouraged me to dress like the woman I wanted to become rather than the woman I was at the time, which was a young, slightly insecure California transplant just finding her footing. While changing the way I dressed may seem like a small detail, it was a defining moment for me. As a twentysomething I hadn't yet found my voice, but I did find a way in which I could let my voice be heard. I saw how fashion gave a voice to those around me and I wanted it to do that for me, too. I quickly learned that what I chose to put on my body and how I chose to carry myself could speak volumes without my having to open my mouth to speak at all.

As is the case for many New York newbies hoping to work in the industry, my first job at a fashion label was in the mailroom. Although I was literally on the basement level at the bottom of the ladder, I made a conscious effort every day to dress like I was on the cusp of being promoted to president. While this was partly because I genuinely enjoyed the way looking put together and polished when I stepped out the door every morning made me feel, it was also largely influenced by the fact that I knew dressing this way would be a professional way to come to work and a way to earn the respect I knew I wanted and needed if I wanted to excel. The mailroom was anything but glamorous, but that did not stop me from bringing out my inner boss lady while I was sorting the mail.

Today, when hiring for my company, I look for someone coming from the same mind-set. Not only do I want a well-qualified, hardworking individual, but I also want someone who takes the time to respect herself and the environment around her. The key to successfully pulling this off is to look equal parts smart, strong, and sexy. Yes—sexy, in the workplace. There is nothing wrong with allowing your femininity to come across at work, as long as your strength is shown at the same time. For me, our sexuality is equal to our femininity. The word "sexuality," unfortunately, has a negative connotation when applied to how one dresses, especially when applied to work wear. However, women are made up of many qualities, and there is nothing wrong with showcasing them if we want to, as long as it's in a controlled, thoughtful way. This is done in an effortless manner by many of the women I'd call my muses. They incorporate predetermined feminine elements into their overall look and always balance those with masculine elements as well.

For interviews, I suggest leaving the mini purses at home and arriving at meetings with a structured bag that mimics a briefcase. From a superior's standpoint, your intelligent piece quite possibly contains important files and datebooks (it might also contain a pair of flats or heels that is neatly disguised). It isn't enough to put together a distinguished outfit. As an employer, I want to hear and see that you mean business, and came with ideas as well as solutions. Another thing I look for during the interview process is the ability to not only dress the part, but be the part. This may sound like a vague ambition, but the energy a truly confident employee projects is tangible to those around him or her, and inspires a sense of trust and respect. Sophistication doesn't end with a smart outfit. Know everything you can about the great restaurants, books, and current affairs that are making headlines, and you will appear well rounded, well educated, well informed, aware, and therefore an invaluable addition to the team. The topics you choose to invest your time and energy into learning on a deeper level should be authentically interesting and inspiring to you, even if they're beyond the boundaries of your current world. Whether you know about cities, countries, hotels you frequent (or, in most cases, wish to frequent)—there's nothing wrong with knowing the best but not being able to afford it . . . yet. The right shoe will get your foot in the door, but your intelligence and how you share it are what will keep you inside. Cultivating a deep, passionate, and comprehensive knowledge of a variety of topics will do wonders for building your confidence and contributing to your value as an employee. Do the research to not just dress the part, but speak the part as well. Putting this extra work in is how you not only look like the role you want to embody, but actually are the role. And never underestimate the power of simply being as helpful as possible—whether it's in your job description or not, do it. Go above and beyond in all areas and you'll work your way up the ladder and out of the mailroom. It is how I finally left the mailroom and was trusted to run other divisions.

THE CREATION

When women officially joined the non-domestic workforce in the 1890s, blouses quickly became the new aprons. Throughout the decades, and at present, blouses have been the standard for office wear and beyond. While they have become a common uniform, they do not have to be boring—in fact, they can be anything but. With a plethora of different fabrics, shapes, and styles, the little white blouse can be one of the most versatile pieces in your closet, simultaneously convenient yet stylish, and when made well, it can be just as comfortable as a tee shirt. Wearing one of these tops tucked into a pencil skirt, tailored trousers, or even a pair of denim jeans lends any ensemble classic strength and elegance.

While the white blouse comes in many different fabrics, I tend to lean toward synthetic blends because they frame my body well without being easily wrinkled. Although many people tend to not care for blended fabrics, I seek them out specifically for travel or work because I can't afford the time in the morning to iron and steam, and I definitely don't have the luxury of doing a costume change at various points throughout the day if I wrinkle. One excellent way to avoid this issue altogether is to opt for non-wrinkle fabrics when and where it counts: work wear. I consistently and unfailingly feel confident and comfortable wearing an easy, elegant white blouse to work, and to me, that's the best foundation to build from.

Considering your shape and what is most flattering for your body type is a key element to looking and feeling your best. I recommend scaling down a size for a more fitted, feminine look, balancing the masculine structure of a blazer with a sexier-fitting blouse. A wise alternative way to wear the blouse is to seek out an oversized option in a softer fabric and pair it with a more slender pant, which exemplifies a refined look with a less serious approach.

A seemingly minor detail that makes a big difference is the collar. The collar of a blouse can definitely determine the vibe of your outfit. For example, a voluminous bow at the neck replaced with a turned-up collar instantly takes a look from romantic to preppy. No matter which way you prefer to wear it, a beautiful blouse always ties an outfit together and says smart and sophisticated.

THE INSPIRATION

Finding inspiration to pull from is a regular practice for me. I like to set aside at least twenty minutes when I can to seek out information that sparks my creativity. I don't only limit my search to style sources, either—I examine the areas of news, food, art, and music, too. Luckily, pursuing information and influence is easy in this digital age. We are able to almost instantly and effortlessly find people and brands to inspire us, and we can keep close tabs on them by following their social media accounts. I encourage you to reserve time for yourself to seek out inspiration the same way you would a facial, a massage, or a meeting. The reason behind the importance and power of this time goes back to the vision board. If you keep feeding yourself visuals of what you praise, those things become part of your life. They just do. What most bloggers and influencers have in common is that they are constantly reminding us of what they are attracted to, and that attracts us to them. That point is key to both whom we choose to follow and why we admire them, and also why they have a career doing what they love. They give consistent content to their consumer that is authentic, informed, and influenced by a deep passion for their field. To have a regular, cohesive style is to be constant in what we do day to day. Setting aside that inspiration time for yourself is paramount to cultivating your own consistency and creating a more definitive identity.

When it comes to dressing in a way that exemplifies smarts and strength, one woman I choose to channel is the perpetually stunning Diane Sawyer. Diane is a loyalist to clean lines and classic cuts, yet still remains in my eyes incredibly attractive and effortless in her femininity. From a quintessential white blouse to a black off-shoulder dress, she is consistently polished, structured, and spot-on. Diane's personal style is known to be monochromatic, usually in natural hues, although she plays with a pop of color from time to time. She has an undeniable ability to successfully capture the spotlight; her clothes never upstage her. Styling has always felt like an extraordinary experience, because rather than focusing on the pieces I'm working with, in the end I only see her and not one of my dresses. In fact, I don't really see the dress at all. Not even the jewelry she wears outshines her. This, I believe, is the ultimate goal of designing and styling. Her style speaks to her accomplishments, how happy she is, and the way she makes people feel. Even if she were not the incomparable, successful woman we all know her to be, the way she carries herself in the clothing she selects would still garner her an elevated level of respect and admiration. What I take from Diane's style is a straightforward lesson: when it comes to your wardrobe, choose pieces that possess the same attributes you wish to embody as a woman. For me, those features include intelligence, grace, and the courage to be beautiful. Some of us feel we must dumb down our looks and our sexuality in order to not make others feel uncomfortable, in order to advance in careers filled with men in upper-level positions. That is simply not true. Diane, for me, is proof that it is not only possible, but preferable to let your true self shine in all your potential. She is at the top of her game, one could say, while still being beautiful, sexy, strong, and feminine.

From the beginning of my career there has been one common denominator on each mood board from every collection I've designed: Carine Roitfeld. The epitome of Parisian chic, Carine—former editor in chief of *Vogue Paris,* founder and current editor in chief of *CR Fashion Book*—is also a muse, model, and mother. Her French style can best be described as perfectly tousled with passion-filled sex appeal. A typical Carine moment might consist of slightly messed hair, charcoal-smudged lined eyes, and an undone collared shirt beneath layers of gold necklaces. The way she pulls it all together, she might as well be donning a spectacular ball gown, because it commands the same regard. The way she constructs a look and the way she wears it become far more interesting than the garments she is actually wearing, because she presents a whole package that tells a story of who she is as a person. To me, the tale she's telling through her fashion says she's a very busy woman with intriguing places to get to and interesting things to say. She appears effortless but meaningful, thoughtful yet mysterious. Carine inspires me to achieve the same storytelling status she does through both my collections and my personal style.

THE PHILOSOPHY

The benefit of having a solid style in the workplace isn't limited to how it can make you appear put together. How we dress affects the way we believe in ourselves and hold ourselves, and as a result, this profoundly impacts how others believe in us as well. Establishing a distinct personal style helps us get closer to actually looking our best because it affords us the confidence to feel like we already have it all together. Even on the days when you perhaps have a fight with your lover or a difficult time getting the children to school, or when you are absolutely crazed at work, you can straighten yourself up on the outside and it will have a profound effect on how you feel on the inside. We might not ever truly have every single duck in a row, and that's the reality of life. What matters is that we make the effort, knowing we and the people we treasure around us who share our life are worthy of that effort.

95

———

HAVING IT ALL (IN YOUR CLOSET):
Key Pieces Every Working Woman Should Own

Today's power suit is minimal but robust. My working uniform is based around pieces that frame my body, show strength in my shoulders, and narrow my waist, while speaking in a way that is true to my personality and personal strengths.

DAY TO NIGHT

In an effort to balance our personal and professional lives, we often run short on time. I'm always trying to squeeze more into each and every hour of the day. The best way to minimize the juggle and maximize your ability to be both present and prepared in all settings is to select an outfit that can seamlessly transition from corner office to cocktails, so to speak. One of my favorite items that I design and often wear to work is the jumpsuit. The reason why it works is because of the power of the singular item to elongate; a one-piece can take you from your first meeting at work to looking as if you are the one most likely to know where the party to be at is. Like a blazer, if it has long sleeves, it frames your body while giving you a strong shoulder, and with a few minor adjustments in accessories and button placement you can also become unapologetically strong and sexy for that evening's event. While it may not be the most conventional choice, I'll consistently opt for the jumpsuit before I'll opt for the little black dress. Both are reliable, classic staples, but the jumpsuit lends a bit more personality and style to the overall aesthetic, in my opinion, and the slightly unexpected look comes across as fresh and modern. I've worn a jumpsuit to the Met Ball, the White House, and even a parent-teacher conference. It's my go-to because it goes everywhere, is easy, and is universally flattering.

My turtleneck tip is one that usually surprises my friends and clients, but it's also one they end up loving the most. If a dress is best suited for my after-hour plans, I'll wear a strapless dress and pair it with a thin, tight turtleneck underneath. It tones down most strapless dresses and makes them instantly more work appropriate. It also extends spring/summer dresses to year-round wardrobe staples. Once the sun goes down, the strapless dress can easily be transformed by simply removing the turtleneck and swapping accessories. Removing sheer black hosiery and adding fishnet stockings with an open-toe, lace-up heel is a provocative way to make a subtle, yet powerful ensemble change. Tuck a clutch into your briefcase-inspired handbag before you leave for the office in the morning so you have the perfect accouterment with you when you're ready to go in the evening.

TROUSERS

Regardless of any chaos that might be happening around or within me, I feel much more put together on the outside, and ultimately on the inside, when I put on a pair of perfect-fitting trousers. Many well-tailored pairs of trousers have a slight stretch in them, and for that reason, I would describe them as my personal form of publicly appropriate undercover sweatpants.

Buying the right pair of trousers for your body type might seem like a daunting chore. But finding the perfect pants doesn't have to drain your time, energy, or wallet. I have a few key recommendations that can make the process far less painful. There are three different versatile and universally flattering trousers I go to and recommend becoming staples in your wardrobe, too:

1. **Leather leggings.** These iconic pants provide a cool, edgy vibe to an outfit while maintaining a polished and professional overall look. In fact, leather leggings are so comfortable that I not only wear them to the office with blazers but also pair them with cardigans and travel in them, too. They can be mixed and matched with so many different tops, depending on whether you're dressing up or down. They're well worth investing in because season after season, these pants are consistently in style yet are as comfortable as jersey leggings.

2. **High-waist trousers** in crepe are another key item. Crepe is a silky fabric that does not have to be 100 percent natural. I like the semi-synthetic mixed crepe because the fabric is durable, thick, and does not wrinkle (as I've mentioned previously, this is key for a crisp, clean look that lasts all day and when traveling); it wears well as it allows for stretch. A major difference between this fabric and 100 percent cotton or silk is that most 100 percent fabrics don't allow for that important bit of stretch, and they wrinkle terribly. Although there are many beautiful articles of clothing that are made of 100 percent cotton, linen, or silk, they're not the fabrics I would suggest as go-tos to feel good about your body while you're running errands, spending quality time with your family, and so on.

The key to finding a crepe trouser that will look good and hold you in is to run your fingers across the fabric. If it feels thin, then I say admire it in the store but leave it. The thin fabric will show every little thing and that's not a good thing for your staple uniform trousers. A thicker crepe fabric with a touch of texture is a much better choice. The combination of elements covers flaws, and feels and looks super on the female form.

The high-waist style is also incredibly flattering, simultaneously elongating your torso, covering the tummy, and lengthening your legs. The general rule of thumb is, the higher the waist, the longer the leg. The versatility of this staple also makes it a must-have: the leg can be cut wide or worn cigarette-style, pegged at the ankle. Whether you're five feet ten or five feet two, chances are you'll have to have these pants hemmed to fit your frame. Tuck a tee shirt or blouse into these high-waist trousers and you'll look and feel polished and empowered.

3. **Boyfriend trousers.** These share many elements of and fit like a pair of boyfriend jeans. They sit lower on the waist and have a relaxed, straight fit from the hip to the cuff. Unlike high-waist trousers, the fabric that I believe works best here is either a wool blend with slight stretch or a heavier 100 percent wool for cooler months. Both are fantastic because they are heavy and do not hug the low hips, or the "ears" of a woman's body, as I call them. They are flattering and comfortable, two great self-esteem boosters. I know that any time I'm not feeling my best and I'm focusing on my insecurities, great things rarely happen. Conversely, when I

embrace and emit positivity, good things seem to flow my way much more easily. A pair of wool-blend boyfriend trousers are an addicting conduit to this look-good, feel-good mind-set.

JEWELRY

Wearing a variety of jewelry is an easy way of expressing your personality in the workplace. I usually choose my outfit first and accent it with accessories that complement it, but I make exceptions for truly special pieces of jewelry. When I have a statement piece I adore, I dress around the jewelry by building my outfit around that item. For example, I adore grand-scale necklaces. I'll wear them to upgrade a uniform outfit or a tee and denim, elevate a turtleneck, and offer some life peeking out from under a trench. The wardrobe upgrade options are endless.

I also aim to let my earrings express my personality. I like to look for different pairs of studs, ear jackets, and ear crawlers in my jewelry box and choose ones that weren't meant to go as a pair but, when put together, tell a story for that day. I also like to let large-scale earrings tell a different type of style story, though they are usually saved for evening events, since I don't want them to be too heavy or uncomfortable and distracting at the office unless they are fun, light costume clip-ons.

Over the years, Bea Valdes, my go-to large-scale jewelry designer, has given me invaluable tips and advice when it comes to selecting the right accessories. I appreciate that her pieces work in a way that can look polished and chic on a casual weekend or can be worn to somewhere special as a major moment. Bea and I both believe that a statement necklace not only makes a statement in jewelry, but also creates a statement about who the woman wearing the jewelry is. It should be consistent with your personal style. Our goals, confidence, and sense of self are expressed not only in what we say each day, but also in our posture and clothing choices, and extend through our jewelry choices. To me, that is another tremendous way to tell the world how to perceive and feel about us without ever having to open our mouths or utter a word. At the end of the day, style is all about telling the story of who you are and who you want to be in the world. By dressing the way you want to be thought of and treated, you're inviting that respect and admiration into your life.

Jewelry is such a personal preference; I encourage you to choose jewelry that embodies the essence of your personality. It is a wonderful way to exude tenacity and grace, to show the world who you are by wearing your personality—literally—on your sleeve. Jewelry is most flattering and will help you to feel your best when balanced with your outfits and when it speaks to who you are and what makes you uniquely you. One of my favorite rings is a large-scale cowrie shell ring by Mesi Jilly. She collects shells from islands she travels to, drills finger holes in them, encrusts them in semiprecious stones, and names each one based on the locale that inspired it; the end result is both stunning and graphic. I also collect shells personally, so the ring is an extension of what I love and the nature that moves me. I get so many compliments on it as well as questions about its origin. I think of it as a visual piece that represents my life on my hand, offering an authentic, eye-opening look at what makes me tick and what moves me.

101

A simple gold or silver choker can add significance and strength to the slight area of your neck. Priests and clergy wear a distinct collar close to their necks, and the area is one that signifies status and influence. A subtle statement in that area, such as a gold or silver collar necklace, can also be a powerful one. Another mainstay in my jewelry rotation is a thin gold choker. It quickly gives my uniform of a blazer and V-neck sweater a refined strength.

Jewelry does not have to be dramatic to be impactful. In my mind, pieces of jewelry have to be statements that are thoughtful and well placed. Again, knowing yourself and your likes and dislikes will get you there. Using as many visual aids as possible and being willing to experiment through trial and error are key to uncovering your jewelry style identity.

When it comes to identifying your personal jewelry style, first see what types of pieces attract you. What do you lean toward in different stores and online boutiques, and in magazines? That will help you to identify and shape your preferences. Also, it's integral to know what makes you feel comfortable and happy and allows you to exude your spirit. Don't be concerned with trends or what other people are wearing or think you should be wearing. Try on different styles to see which types of earrings and necklaces frame your face and flatter you, and add from there. For example, when I wear my hair in a tight, low bun I love to wear my Indian chandelier earrings with a simple outfit. I do not like wearing them when my hair is long and down because it creates too much distraction. Building the right look is all about incorporating balance, so if you're going for eye-catching accessories, tone down your look everywhere else.

Selecting the Right Statement Jewelry

TIPS FROM BEA VALDES

Bea Valdes is an award-winning, world-renowned luxury goods and accessories designer whom I have been a fan of for years. She is also kind enough to offer her advice on making smart jewelry choices.

I would recommend a woman selects the pieces that really reflect her character. That is, not too much "of the moment" or just on trend. If she can imagine that it is something she could wear next season, and ten years down the line, then the piece is for her.

I would definitely suggest considering the quality of the piece, the way that it is made, and, even if it uses humble materials, whether they are designed well and deeply.

Again, it should be not just a statement, but part of one's signature look.

It is, as they say, not just about the jewelry but the woman who wears it.

Every woman should own a statement ring, a pair of earrings, and a necklace, but probably not worn all together! And of the three, the necklace is probably the most memorable piece.

Find what you are comfortable in, which cuts and fit flatter you, and build solidly from there.

Do not be too concerned with trends, as they are secondary to your style.

Build a wardrobe around these strengths first, as the key is to invest in how comfortable and confident you are, both in your clothes and in your own skin.

Personal style comes to fruition when a customer begins to refer to a piece as her *own* jewelry; she sees it as something designed by me but ultimately the piece really has found its owner. It's not just a statement piece, but a signature piece, something that is an extension of one's character.

Most of my pieces are quite bold or unique, but I find women to be the same.

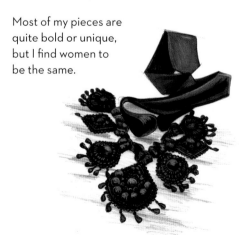

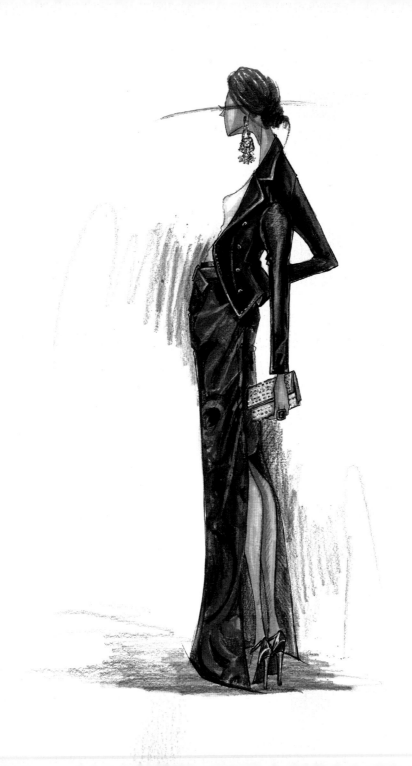

· 6 ·

BEING THE WELL-DRESSED GUEST

KINDNESS IS ALWAYS FASHIONABLE

*Before you
leave the house,
remove one piece.*

—COCO CHANEL

I have loved fashion my whole life but for many years was not able to afford my favorite pieces from the designers I admired. The moment I was able to afford the clothes I wanted, I went a bit overboard.

In fact, when I was finally able to just go for it and splurge on the designer clothes I'd been drooling over for so many years, I went slightly off track and got insanely "experimental." Looking back on the experience, I liken it to being exceptionally hungry—borderline famished—and finally having the opportunity to sit down for a really hearty meal. I felt like I had to consume every single morsel on the table in haste without using utensils or stopping to even take a breath. The opportunity to indulge was so overwhelming that I did just that. When I was finally able to become a customer in the boutiques where once I could only window-shop, I put all of my money into one single outfit rather than thoughtfully spreading out my funds. No single moment epitomizes this poorly thought-out strategy more than one of my first big red carpet events. Years ago I went to the VH1 Fashion Awards show dressed head to toe in designer labels. It wasn't how I thought one should dress for such an occasion, but I understand now what I was feeling at the time—I compare it to being like an overexcited tourist wearing everything in her suitcase at once. I paired a black-and-silver-beaded Chloé miniskirt with a hot pink Birkin bag and sky-high designer heels. To finish off the over-the-top look, I accessorized with wild earrings that were nearly completely obscured behind my overly styled bouffant hair. Thankfully, I at least had the sense to pair the skirt with a simple white men's blouse, so it wasn't total body chaos. However, I had the nerve to tie the simple shirt at my waist, showing off my waistline. At the time, I thought I was actually being wise because the designer blouse was far too short for my frame. I hadn't been able to resist the urge to buy the piece anyway, thinking that if I just knotted it at the waist, it would appear as if I had intentionally styled it to be that short. I wasn't fooling anyone, though, least of all myself. The second I stepped outside the house I felt silly, overdone, and overtly tacky. The uneasiness only escalated the closer I got to the event, and by the time I reached the red carpet, I was undeniably (and I'm sure visibly) uncomfortable. Although it was an unpleasant experience to go through, it became a very important lesson in understanding and internalizing the mantra "Just because you can, does not mean you should." More important than how ridiculous I looked, I *felt* extremely uncomfortable in my own skin, and that feeling looks good on absolutely no one. I did not have a good time that night, and it wasn't because the event was unentertaining. It was because I dressed in a way that I thought others wanted me to dress and not the way I wanted to dress. I learned that night that great style means knowing how to balance comfort and personality, style and grace, and not falling victim to each and every trend and tempting designer item on the rack. Great style is knowing who you are and dressing that way.

Luckily, I had the opportunity to make up for my fashion blunder soon afterward. I was invited to an opening-night dinner for the Tribeca Film Festival. After my disastrous style choices for the VH1 awards, I decided to go in the opposite direction for the opening of the film festival and I dressed true to myself, styled the way I wanted to look and how I felt comfortable. I paired a Ralph Lauren sparkly bolero with a white tank, my favorite pair of vintage men's 501 jeans, and stunning Alaïa sandals. I also wore my hair naturally. No more bouffant blowouts for me. I felt so confident in the end result, knowing the ensemble was not only a true reflection of my own style, but also a comfortable, cool choice for the event I was attending—or any event, quite frankly. The outfit gave the impression that while I took both myself and the event seriously, I was also respectful to the host. I was keeping with my own standards and comfort level that evening. Although I was wearing denim, the way they were styled made them cocktail worthy, and many women in ball gowns came up to me that night and confided, "I wish I'd worn jeans, too!" I looked and felt completely at ease, and that joyful feeling was evident to everyone I came across that night. If the VH1 event was an important lesson in "less is more," then the Tribeca opening night dinner taught me that happiness is the key to creating the best style every time.

THE CREATION

When I received an invitation to the wedding of my friends Kim Kardashian and Kanye West, I immediately knew I wanted to wear a men's tuxedo. And by "men's tuxedo" I literally mean a men's tux. The wedding ceremony was slated to take place in Paris and the reception was taking place at another, undisclosed location, so I knew from the onset that travel would be a necessity. Knowing this couple and the surprises they were capable of, I also considered the possibility that the international celebration could even involve an additional flight or two or three. Since I knew I likely would not have a lot of time to change while traveling from the ceremony to the reception, it was important to ensure that my garments stayed fresh and neat while en route from one location to another hour after hour, dance after dance. I also considered the fact that I did not want to be toting a lot of luggage to and from airports, country to country. First and foremost, however, the most important detail I wanted to consider was how to feel truly comfortable in my own skin during the event itself; to accomplish this, I always turn to the looks that I know work

110

best for my body and my style preferences. Rather than worrying myself with what everyone else was choosing to wear, I knew it was important for me to wear what I would feel most comfortable in and what would make me feel true to my own taste. This would allow me to be the best, most present guest I could be, and allow me to truly be able to focus on the beautiful occasion, and not be distracted by my own discomfort.

After deciding to wear a tuxedo to the wedding, I went to the men's Saint Laurent store in order to find one that could be easily tailored to accommodate my height and shape. Without much deliberation, I decided to go with a midnight navy suit with a black lapel and black tuxedo stripe down the trouser—midnight and black never fails. Rather than going for an all-black ensemble, I wanted to allow for slight variation and to truly make the look classically me. I asked the store to tailor the tux to fit my measurements. In addition to tightly narrowing the waist, I asked for the ankle to be taken in, in order to accentuate my overall shape and offer a feminine touch; the tailor wisely added a thin, invisible black zipper to the inside of the ankle in order to help me get in and out of the tux with ease. The zipper also served another ingenious purpose, giving me the option to leave the leg unzipped so that I could wear the pants with a variety of different shoes for future events. Underneath the shawl collar jacket, I wore a men's-style white J.Crew shirt. I opted to size down so that the top could accentuate and feminize my frame. This ensured the blouse would fit well under the jacket, and the tighter fit infused the menswear look with a hint of feminine sexuality. To keep the look from being too masculine, I left the blouse practically unbuttoned, in order to reveal just the right amount of my lace underpinnings. Showing a bit of skin when wearing menswear instantly softens an ensemble. I paired the tux with the most seductive Manolos I owned, again to balance. I chose a pair of heels that I had in my closet for a while rather than buying something brand-new, because I knew that the broken-in pair would be comfortable and keep my feet from aching after hours of travel and celebration, not to mention Italian cobblestone, a killer! The clean, structured yet classically compelling look that I wore to the wedding afforded me comfort, confidence, and the ability to focus on the stunning, romantic wedding of friends.

THE INSPIRATION

My brother invited me to join him for a work event he had at the Museum of Modern Art that was extremely important to him, yet after a long, hard day of work, the last thing I felt like doing was going anywhere far from the comfort of my bed. However, I knew I wanted to show support for my brother, who had been unconditionally supportive of me for so many years. The desire to be there for him and to show how much I cared was what eventually motivated me to pull myself together and assemble a look that reflected how proud I truly was to stand by him. That night I chose a sparkly vintage wrap dress that hadn't been tailored to my size and was, in fact, probably two and a half times too big. Rather than let the garment completely consume me, I improvised by adding an unbuttoned men's striped shirt underneath, and wrapped the whole look together with a classic men's brown vintage belt. I threw on yellow oxford men's shoes to ensure that my already tired feet would be completely comfortable for the evening yet not boring, in at least color and shape, and the look was complete. Putting the effort into looking and feeling my best (yet super comfy) transformed my mood and energy level, and I went from wanting to stay home to feeling poised, polished, and ready to take whatever came my way in an effort to support my brother. What made me feel even better that night was the way my brother's eyes lit up when I appeared at MoMA. He did not fail to recognize that I had taken the time and effort to get myself together in order to support him. He loved the outfit and said so immediately upon seeing me. And what I loved was that a small effort on my part to dress up was so appreciated by a loved one. This experience shaped my understanding that when we look and feel our best, it can truly have a profound impact on those around us, particularly our loved ones. It makes others feel good when it's clear that you've gone out of your way for them, because it shows not only the respect you have for yourself, but that you genuinely care about them and want to present your best self for them as well. Getting dressed to the nines doesn't always only affect how we feel about ourselves, sometimes it affects those we care about as well. I know my presence at his event that night demonstrated to my brother how much I value him and care about him, and that I wanted to not only show up, but to be completely present for him and participate in his life by standing by his side and showing my support.

113

THE PHILOSOPHY

When invited to someone's home or party, I consider dressing re-spectfully to be just as important as bringing the host a gift. When attending someone's event, I always consider all of the energy the host put into planning the festivities and I try to match that effort in my attire. I take to heart that the host spent time preparing a space or a meal, or creating an experience for me, and I want to reciprocate the effort and energy in every way I can. One way to try to match that is by putting thought into how I present myself. I consider what I can wear, and what I can do to support the host's endeavors in making the event happen. Whether it is an intimate party or a huge soiree, being respectful to the work done to create the event is some-thing I always keep in mind.

114

    This year I attended a wedding in Malibu with a friend. I knew from a member of the wedding party that the groomsmen would be wearing tuxedos. Because he was not a groomsman and he knew the wedding would be at the beach, my friend assumed that the dress code would be casual. Before the ceremony, my friend told me he planned to wear a linen button-down shirt for a more casual look. I explained to him that men in the wedding party would be wearing tuxedos and that this was a decision the bride and groom had intentionally made when setting the tone for their wedding. I advised him that it was important that as guests, we should dress in a way that was compatible with the decisions they had made when planning the wedding. Whenever I'm invited to participate in a life event as momentous as a wedding, I always devote a significant amount of thought to the couple who is getting married and carefully consider all the things I know about the bride's and groom's personalities. What are some of their likes and dislikes? What type of attire would they appreciate we wear, and how would what we choose to wear enhance the tone of one of the most important days that will last in their memories? Thinking about a color the couple loves, or incorporating their heritage into your look, is also a kind way to participate in a respectful yet celebratory fashion. Being gracious and conscientious in your wardrobe is just as important as your positive, joy-filled attitude at someone else's significant event.

When you don't know the dress code, it's always best to play it safe. How you style your hair and the accessories you choose can be key. Creating a clean palette with your hair by going for a low ponytail or bun creates a conservative base that will give you carte blanche to wear just about anything. You can wear an LBD or even a jumpsuit, but, as always, consider how you will accessorize. I personally like having the option of being slightly overdressed versus being underdressed, because I know I'm more likely to project confidence and poise when I err on the side of formal as opposed to casual. However, you can get away with underdressing if your hair, makeup, and accessories are sophisticated enough and successfully elevate your look without being distracting. For some occasions, you can get away with the most basic staples, as long as you wear them well. For example, when accessorized correctly, a nice-fitting pair of jeans with a white blouse can be a very sophisticated look that can be worn for many types of occasions.

When all else fails and you don't know what to wear, the best strategy is to just channel style icon Audrey Hepburn or someone similar who is inspiring to you. A crisp white shirt with a sweater over it, capris, and ballet flats—these simple yet elegant clothing items can go a long way in many different fashion settings and situations. Clean and classic ensembles are always appropriate and will make you feel comfortable in your own skin. Rather than going overboard like I did at the VH1 event, think about how Audrey paired her classic, clean, simple style with a heavy dose of respect and kindness, and you can't go wrong.

———

STEPPING IT UP WHEN STEPPING OUT

Dressing with elegance doesn't have to mean dressing in a way that makes you feel uncomfortable. And just because you're attending a dressy event does not mean you have to wear a dress. If a more traditional ensemble just isn't your thing, there's no reason you have to compromise your comfort for the sake of convention. Here are some alternative ways to step it up when stepping out.

FLOOR-SWEEPING SKIRTS

I wear these a lot because they are so versatile. The skirt can be the focal point of the ensemble, or you can wear one that makes a more subtle statement and pair it with a turtleneck and a statement necklace. One key detail to consider is to make sure the length of the skirt is appropriate for your height and to get the skirt hemmed if it is too long for your frame. Another option is to try turning a floor sweeper into a maxi-skirt by shortening the length to just above the ankle or toward the lower part of the calf for a midi length. A glimpse of skin at the ankle gives a very elegant, elongating effect.

TUXEDO PANTS

I can't tell you how much I adore these pants. You can achieve a balance pairing a solid, masculine pant with a softer, feminine fit. Tuxedo pants are tremendous basic staples, because you can wear them the way you'd normally wear a capri pant or you can opt for a longer length. I love the array of options tuxedo pants provide, and the fact that you can almost always find a style that works for your particular tastes, body type, and event needs. For a casual look, I pair tuxedo pants with flats, a tee shirt, and a cardigan. For a more elegant look, wear tuxedo pants with a men's button-down shirt over a beaded tank top paired with a strappy high-heeled sandal.

117

SILK SHORTS

A blazer and tucked-in blouse paired with silk shorts are a classic variation of the uniform blazer look. Wearing silk shorts with a high-heeled oxford and tights or a ballerina flat provides that perfect balance of femininity and masculinity when you incorporate all the right elements: a powerful blazer, a softer short, a tailored shoe, and a men's-style watch. The right length of short allows one to show off a pair of toned legs, but sculpted calves and slender thighs are not required in order to pull off a pair of shorts. There are so

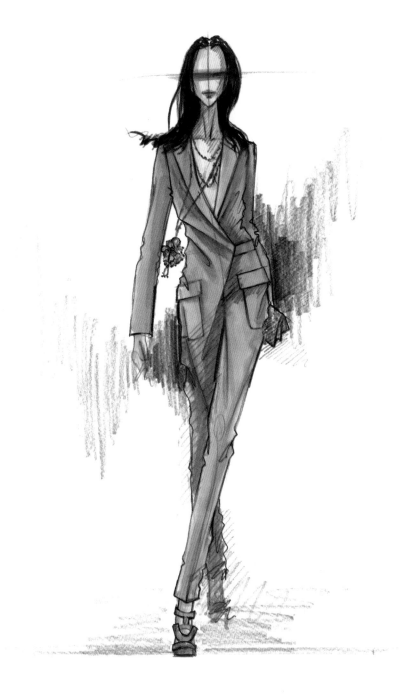

many types and styles of tights on the market that can enhance the legs of women who don't have time to be constant gym bunnies. Try the trick many singers use onstage by wearing nude or black fishnets, which cover all the flaws while providing just the right amount of sexiness and allure. Or try a sheer black color with a thin seam up the back of the leg for a classic sense of seductiveness. There are so many options to play up the parts you love while camouflaging the areas that may not be your favorite. Thanks to the endless possibilities, shorts in varying shapes and lengths can be a smart staple for everyone.

JUMPSUITS

Among my favorite pieces, a jumpsuit elongates every body and flatters many different shapes. For more casual moments, wear a loose-fitting silk jumpsuit cinched at the waist with a vintage belt. For more formal occasions, a long-sleeved strong-shoulder jumpsuit can lend just the right amount of sophisticated style. I also love the look of a strapless jumpsuit worn with a thin, tight turtleneck and a men's blazer thrown over the shoulders, paired with a statement shoe for the evening.

SCARVES

This is one of the ways I can instantly up the sophistication factor or completely change the look of any outfit. Loosely wrapping a scarf several times around your neck can quickly soften a structured blazer and tone down the edginess of an outfit while adding that cool bohemian vibe. Alternatively, letting the middle of the scarf sit at the base of your neck and allowing the ends to flow behind you can add an instant dramatic flair, à la Grace Kelly circa 1950. A constant for me is wearing a long scarf around my neck and tying a belt around my waist, on the outside of the scarf (see image on page 174)—it allows for an added dimension and creates an element of individual poise in the outfit, plus it makes you look like an editor, which is cool. A scarf can also mean the difference between feeling less than glamorous and feeling completely at ease, easily transforming a bad hair day into a style statement. Using a brightly colored scarf as a turban can give you a sense of distinctly personal style—you just need to find a good friend who knows how to tie one for you! The style also works well as a headband turban if you can't quite commit to the full turban look—think Sharon Stone in *Casino*.

120

"The amen of nature is always a flower."
—OLIVER HOLMES

Flowers are a gracious, traditional gift that just about everyone is thankful to receive. Whether you're hosting an at-home celebration or are invited as a guest to a soiree, providing beautiful blooms is a thoughtful way to say thank you; it's a message that I know I personally always appreciate. Eric Buterbaugh is well-known for being the premier florist to fashion and floral lovers who cherish all things that blossom. He also happens to be a dear friend who always comes equipped with exceptional advice for designing with flowers in ways that will inspire the space around you. Eric comes from a fashion-

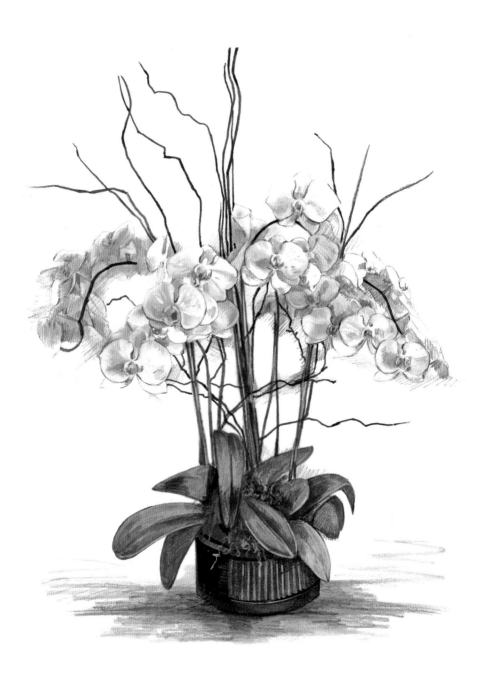

based background, so it's not surprising that his guidelines for floral arrangements are very similar to what works when it comes to style. Flowers are the natural luxury accessory, beautifully and dependably enhancing both professional and personal spaces.

The general rule when working with flowers is that less is more: "Whether you are getting your flowers at a flower market or the grocery store, one simple rule to live by is to not make the arrangement too complicated," Eric advises. "Sometimes people get it into their heads that the more different flowers that they incorporate into a bouquet, the better . . . I tend to disagree. Masses of any type of flower always look better to me." Rather than stocking up on every flower variety in the store, Eric believes it's best to pick a distinctive direction and to follow through on that theme to create a clean, cohesive, beautiful blend. "I always suggest coming up with one color palette or just using a mass of one type of flower," he says. "Therefore you avoid creating a fruit salad and instead are dealing with a single ingredient, a chic arrangement. People need to stop making everything so complicated when it comes to florals. The easier the better, in my opinion."

Draw the eyes upward: "A trick I use is to find vases and vessels to put the flowers into that are not clear—this way you don't have to see the stems or the water," Eric says. Rather than opting for the traditional see-through container, try going for something that will keep all the attention on the beautiful blooms, not the stems below. "In my flower studio, we leaf line the vases to hide the stems, but if you have a vase that is ceramic or has a design where the stems are hidden, that is always a great way to make the flowers look fresh and clean."

Flowers are the perfect accessory, regardless of the event: "I think that everyone will agree that the florals are the icing on the cake to every event or environment," Eric says. "They are a luxury that everyone can enjoy and they always enhance the look and feel of any space."

123

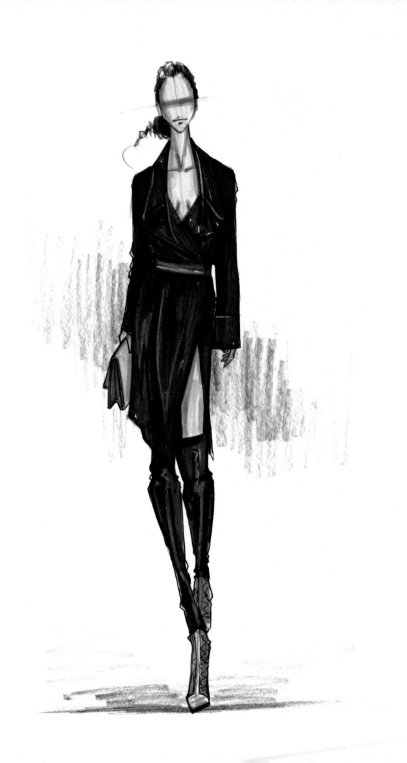

· 7 ·

NOT ALL
SEXY IS
ACTUALLY
SEXY

*Instead of going in
the direction that
a lot of the women
singers are going in
(revealing), I'll be
very sexy under
18 pounds of chiffon
and lace and velvet…
I will have mystique.*

—STEVIE NICKS

D ressing for attention gets a bad rap. In my mind, there is nothing inherently wrong with styling yourself in a manner intended to draw interest. If receiving accolades for your efforts reinforces your confidence, and makes you happy, then by all means go for it.

"Dressing for attention" does not necessarily mean putting it all out there. Is it only attention you're seeking? The sexiest looks are the ones that conjure mystique, intrigue, and challenge, leaving something to the imagination of the viewer or your audience. By strategically revealing and concealing different areas on the body, you create an air of mystery that's actually much more enticing than an all-out exhibition. A hint of skin is enough to draw people in, the same way a hint of an impossibly intriguing conversation pulls in your audience.

The power of suggestion is far more influential than one may realize. Just the subtle implication of sensuality is enough to provoke people's imaginations and intrigue more effectively than blatant sexuality. The media often gets this wrong, unfortunately, and in turn skews our own perception of sex appeal. The wardrobe staples of my favorite classic film starlets—skirts with just the right amount of slit, off-the-shoulder blouses, waist-cinching gowns—exude a sense of control, intelligence, and a knowing, willing, intentional participation in cultivating sexiness. These women weren't just objects to be ogled—they used their clothes as tools to enact their sexuality and entice their audience on their terms. They called the direction. That empowerment is crucial to creating an authentically enticing style, and to becoming a cool, confident, commanding presence.

The real key to sexiness is suggesting there's more than meets the eye. That goes for the overall aesthetic and the implied meaning behind it. On the literal level, exposing just your décolletage and concealing the rest conjures up curiosity about what's not being shown (far sexier than showing too much). On the deeper level, selectively revealing certain body parts and keeping the rest under wraps brings the attention back to you—and you're more than your body, beauty, or clothes; you are a soul. What we present to the world on the outside is important (it is, after all, the main message of this book!), but the exterior packaging is just the way you radiate your inner intellect, spirit, and humanity. Exhibit your value and gifts in a way that reaches beyond just the physical, and others will follow suit. It certainly isn't necessary to stay completely buttoned up (what fun would that be?), but be thoughtful about your choices when deciding on an attention-getting outfit and consider reevaluating the kind of attention you're truly after.

THE CREATION

One of my first jobs working outside of retail was in the early nineties. The assignment was to style an up-and-coming female rapper.

She'd recently had a big hit and I was hired to create a memorable look for the song's video. At the time, I was working primarily for start-up magazines and taking on other entry-level jobs as a way to build my portfolio while working a day job in retail to pay the bills. The styling job felt like a big deal and a significant opportunity outside of what I normally did. I wanted to affect her look and influence the artist and everyone at her label with what I believed true sexiness was. In my head, I was already envisioning future jobs styling her and other women, and I needed to execute this first opportunity perfectly.

After a short time agonizing over what I'd present to her, someone known as much for her sexiness as for her distinct sound, I decided on something made with precision-sharp rigor, something sophisticated and something I would LOVE to wear. An outfit that would have viewers thinking about her, in her absence, not just in their presence. A great ensemble can do just that, so I borrowed a beautiful oxblood turtleneck, a sleek leather pencil skirt, and matching oxblood heels. The pieces were crisp, structured, and impeccably crafted. This artist was just on the brink of stardom and hadn't quite made it big, therefore pulling the items was a major challenge. The all-Gucci ensemble was typically reserved for established celebrities, and I was a newbie in the styling world. Somehow, I pulled it off, and I arrived on set excited to see how the impeccable garments would look on my client and on camera.

When the rapper stepped out of her dressing room, I thought she looked phenomenal. The tight cranberry turtleneck and matching buttery leather skirt to the knee accentuated her curves but left

129

just enough to the imagination. The look exuded a whip-smart conviction that I considered incredibly sexy, because it empowered and enabled the wearer to actually *feel* sexy, not just look it.

While I was thrilled with how my carefully put-together outfit looked on my client, the expression on her face suggested she felt otherwise. To my surprise, she wasn't just indifferent about the look—she was actually quite upset. She wanted me to dress her in something far more revealing and overtly sexual, and to make matters worse, the director agreed with her. I understand the inspiration behind her intention; at the time, women in rap videos were almost exclusively wearing brightly colored fur boleros with too-tight bikini tops or micro bandage dresses. She felt that to stay relevant and keep climbing her way to the top, she needed to go head-to-head with her competition. She didn't feel hot or confident in the outfit I provided, and there was no convincing her otherwise, even though I knew she looked powerful, tough, and like a total badass. My goal coming into the job was to make her look her best and to help her create a look that was both commanding and subtly racy. In my eyes, the look I'd selected put the ball in her court, steering the video's concept toward empowering women and away from objectification. Unfortunately, the rapper wasn't the only one disappointed in the toned-down look. The males in charge were also anticipating a video vixen to purr into the camera while pouring champagne down her string bikini. The last thing they wanted was the sight of a slick, empowered female looking equal parts smart and desirable. I was dismissed on the spot, mid-shoot. I was devastated, but my convictions were not completely shaken by the experience. I was certain that music label would never hire me again for that type of work, yet I felt good in my decision to not dress women like sex objects and to stand up for the ideals I had. I'd unintentionally burned a bridge and compromised my career, but I had my pride and that was something I was born with and raised with, and that to me was more important than a career doing something I did not believe in. A dose of stubbornness paired with good intent can go a long way.

THE INSPIRATION

To my delight and surprise, a few months after the incident, I was hired to work for the same team, who were in the process of founding a clothing company. They may not have wanted me to dress their video vixens again, but they wanted me to join forces with them to dress their consumer: real women. They wanted my vision for style, which they were able to see on the video set, to play a significant part in the creation of their women's line. While my vision for their rapper wasn't one that resonated with the group at the time of the video, they recognized the far-reaching potential this vision had for a larger demographic of women. On set, they'd been intent on reproducing the tried-and-true (but, in my opinion, stale and objectifying) formula for female sexiness. In their new venture, they aspired to appeal to real women in the real world. The style I had created on set hadn't fit the bill that day, but they knew it could work in the right context. Now the same men who had let me go for my out-of-the-box perspective and unwavering commitment to my principles wanted my input and involvement in their new endeavor.

The opportunity was one I'd certainly wanted for years and worked hard and patiently for until it presented itself. Although I never doubted or regretted the choices I made that day for the video shoot, the lesson did not come full circle for a while. The unforeseen opportunity confirmed for me what until then I only hoped was true: that dressing in a way that imitates and impersonates a false concept of sexiness might be effective for achieving a short-term goal, such as starring in a music video, but dressing in a way that exemplifies a woman's class, elegance, and effortless sensuality draws respect, acclaim, and yes, attention, long-term—a lesson I believed in long before I was actually put to the test.

THE PHILOSOPHY

132

If I learned anything from this experience that I want to impart to you, it's the lesson that sticking to your intentions and upholding your values is the key to success in all areas of life, whether it's professional or personal, internal or external. While it can certainly seem easier to compromise your beliefs in favor of falling in line with the popular vote, it's not a strategy I advocate or believe leads to true triumph in any situation. If sticking to your guns and staying true to yourself means losing an opportunity, stay strong, stay positive, and stay firm in your values, morals, and principles. Being true to yourself is the only path I know of that will ensure bigger and better opportunities will come your way. Putting yourself out into the world in the most authentic way possible attracts the opportunities that are right for you—and those aren't always the ones you *think* are right for you in the moment.

We all have gut feelings and strong convictions about issues we care about. For me, I knew that a blatantly sexualized look was not something I wanted to promote or endorse on set that day, or ever, frankly. I knew that dressing my client in clothes that flattered her figure while suggesting viewers should take note of her brain and her talent, not just her body, would be far more creative, a little bit subversive, and, above all, incredibly alluring. I could have scrambled to assemble a midriff-baring, barely there ensemble in order to keep my job and save face on my first big gig, but I would have been sacrificing my integrity, and that's something I won't do. To this day I am only interested in people who stand up for what they believe, especially when it goes against the grain. Some of the most beautiful things in life do not come without risk.

The complicated and conflicting messages we encounter as women (be sexy! but not too sexy! lean in! but don't strive too much!) can leave you feeling like you're fighting a battle that's unfairly stacked against you. So, write your own rules: Self-love. Self-respect. Self-rule.

It would be easy to just do what's expected of us and act in a way that keeps us under the radar, but where would that lead us? It's daily work to reconnect with your true self, but it's well worth the effort and the risks to speak out and stand up for what you believe. If you're not really sure what that is, it's okay. Start small— identify the topics and issues that interest and inspire you. Is it fashion, politics, art, or cinema? Then examine what the prevailing ideas are in those areas and really think critically about whether or not you agree. It's important to note not to overthink it, however. Think critically and be a thinking person, but know when to let it go and trust yourself. This happens when thinking and trusting yourself—merge all while feeling with your heart. Practice on issues you excel at, where thinking easily becomes knowing and trusting what you know. Pay attention to what that feels like and then try to apply the same principles to issues that are a bit more foreign to you. Do you really endorse that candidate, or are you just voting in a way that falls in line with the direction your family leans? Do you really believe that film was worthy of Best Picture, or do you think the Academy got it wrong? These exercises aren't superficial or small—they help me and they'll help you practice rebuilding your identity and cultivating confidence in all areas of your life.

——————

134

Dressing equal parts powerful and sexy is all about balance.

There's a strange phenomenon that I've observed around specific events and holidays. Every time Halloween comes around or Coachella fever ramps up, women seem to wear less and less clothing and reveal more and more skin. Perhaps unsurprisingly, men seem to generally stay pretty well covered through these milestone moments. Seriously?

Look, I get it—I like sometimes selecting seductive outfits for certain moments as well. Celebrations, festivals, and events always seem like a great excuse to go outside the typical day-to-day closet staples and go for some more extraordinary pieces that remix your typical style. But why does that have to translate to T&A only?

My biggest hope for women is that they step away from the trends and expectations and reconnect with who they are inside. True sexiness is not about skin; it's about internal fire and assuredness, strength and fierceness blended with softness and sensuality. It's not about playing the role of a video vixen in order to please a partner or fulfill a fantasy. It's about finding peace and happiness with who you are despite the thorniness of life, and recognizing that what you want is internal. I understand it's easier said than done—learning to be happy with who you are is probably one of life's biggest challenges, and it doesn't happen overnight. But realizing you have a choice in how you present yourself and how you feel is the first step in that journey. It's life-changing to find out what makes you feel amazing, inside and out.

The key is to choose these items with the intention of fulfilling your needs and desires, not to play dress-up for anyone else.

And when putting together an ensemble that you want to exude sexiness, opting for balance and a "less-is-more" aesthetic is far more appealing than grabbing an extra-small for every item. There's no reason I can't wear a low-cut blouse or short skirt and command the same type of respect I receive when covered up in pants and a blazer. But I'm selective about which pieces I incorporate and why, and I encourage you to be the same. If you legitimately love that crop top, consider skipping the miniskirt. If your shortest shorts are right for the occasion, a flowy top can keep your look balanced while still being youthful. Too much of a good thing simply isn't a good thing, and learning to be discerning and thoughtful about which clothes you wear and which body parts you generously showcase to the world can have a profound impact on your self-esteem, style, and, above all, sexiness.

136

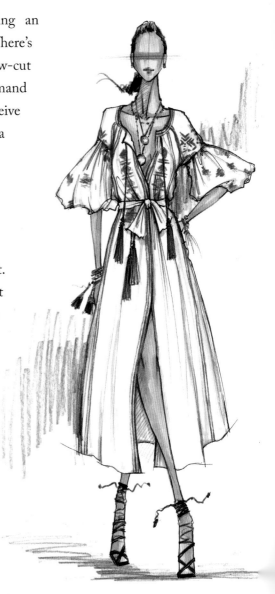

Music Festival

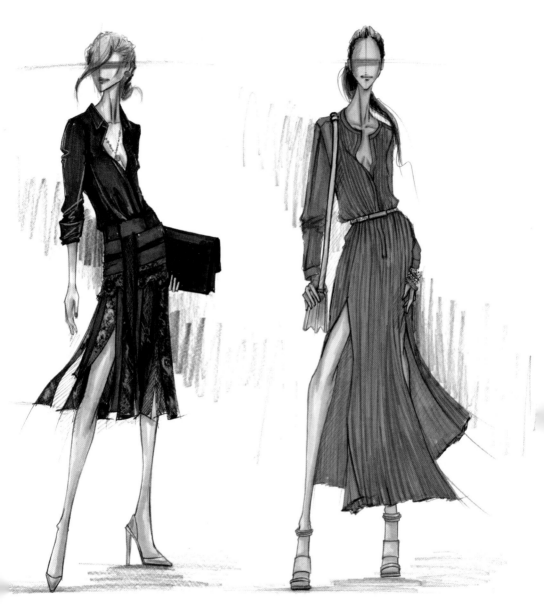

First Date   *Single and (Not Really) Looking*

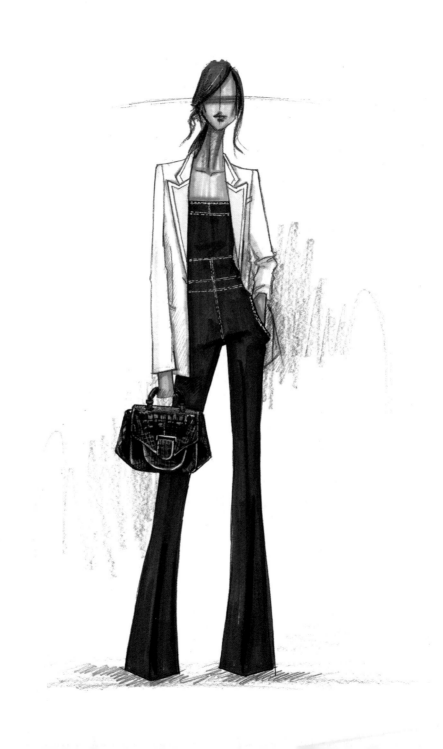

· 8 ·

COMFORTABLY COOL

*Make your wardrobe as
versatile as an actress.
It should be able
to play many roles.*

—JOAN CRAWFORD

As women, we wear many hats and fill a wide variety of roles in a single day, no matter what our official professions are. On my busiest days, I'm not just a designer. I'm a mother, nurse, cleaning lady, driver, entrepreneur, yoga student, amateur chef, and on and on.

I'm up at the crack of dawn getting the kids ready for the day, taking them to school, squeezing in a quick workout, handling business in the office, running errands, picking up the girls, making dinner, attending an event, all the while attempting to be creative on a deadline . . . and eventually collapsing into bed. During my busiest weeks, it's that level of chaos and intensity times seven, rinse and repeat. It would be so effortless and easy to breeze through my day wearing yoga pants, and I understand why so many women do. When I'm constantly on the go and barely have a second to sit down or breathe, even pulling on a proper pair of pants or applying a swipe of mascara seems like a time-sucking chore. I absolutely get the appeal of an all-Lycra-everything outfit on busy days, or a serious moment contemplating whether pajama pants can pass as a bold fashion risk outside the house, but the truth is, dressing in workout clothes for the workday or my personal life on the weekends does nothing for my self-esteem, and can actually take my energy level down a significant number of notches.

We're all guilty of embracing the lazy look out of convenience, lack of time, or, well, laziness. But my thought on this is simply that we can do better than that. Don't get me wrong: I'm not a big believer in the "beauty is pain" philosophy some advocate, and I long for cushy, soft textures and quick, easy options as much as any other woman. Comfort is key to self-confidence, and it isn't just about cutting corners; when you feel comfortable, you project confidence, grace, and sophistication. When you're worrying about the height of your stilettos or gasping for breath beneath a too-tight cocktail dress, it shows. But there's an important distinction here that many women fail to see when assembling their daily outfit. Comfort is important, but comfort is not synonymous with sloppiness.

When you go out into the world, I'm a firm believer that it's important to present the sharpest, brightest, best version of yourself—whether you're shopping for groceries or giving a career-changing presentation. It doesn't matter if you're taking your kids to the playground or working on deadline behind a desk. Wherever you go and whatever you do, it's imperative to channel your highest version of you, and project it out into the world in order to feel the best version of yourself. The truth of the matter is, that's a difficult job to undertake in worn-out stretch pants and your lover's college sweatshirt. If you truly aspire to be successful in all areas of your life, be it business, relationships, motherhood, or friendship, it's important to look and feel the part of a strong, loving, powerful, organized woman. Hitting that stride can be easier than you think.

THE CREATION

Several weeks ago, I had planned some quality time with my fifteen-year-old daughter, Ava. We didn't have grand plans by any means, but in this fast-paced world of schedules and activities, we were overdue for some much-needed bonding and relaxing girl time. After some deliberation back and forth, we decided to peruse the neighborhood bookstore and head to the movies; outside of a day in bed watching Netflix, pretty much the most laid-back Saturday a busy mom could hope for. When getting dressed that morning, I knew I also had a slew of errands to run throughout the day and needed an outfit that was easy, comfortable and functional. But I also wanted to opt for something that Ava would like, too. Considering my options, I landed on a simple, flowing midi dress with leggings, slip-on sneakers, and a black-and-white gingham shirt as a cardigan. The ensemble was a definite step up from workout gear, but it was still completely casual, comfortable, and—I hoped—an outfit that would make my daughter happy as well. When Ava saw me, not only did I get the seal of approval from her, but she wanted to match my mood and "dress up" as well. "Oh, we are looking cute today?" was her exact comment, and she went to change into a similar outfit. What it meant to her was that maybe this was more than running errands; maybe an adventure lay ahead of us, and one did: we ended up at our favorite restaurant by the sea. It made the mommy-daughter day that much more fun, and Ava saw that she was not a passing errand but rather a person whom I wanted to dress up for and look nice for as well. I find my daughters are always happy when I dress up—it not only is fun for them, but lets them know they are just as important as the other events in my life I dress up for. The reality is, they are more important—much more—so I try to show them that through a variety of actions.

In my experience, going for the easiest option isn't a great strategy as the day unfolds. It may seem like a time-saver in the moment you're rushing out the door, but the negative energy it can have on your mood and assurance as the hours pass just isn't worth the minutes spared. With a little thought, you can put together a few exquisite weekend uniforms that are as flattering and just as comfy as your loungewear. I strongly believe that dressing in a way that complements your own style and suits whomever you are spending your day with always pays off. The secret is amassing an arsenal of everyday uniforms that you can throw on and wear with ease, but still look savvy, polished, and put together.

144

THE INSPIRATION

While we dedicate a lot of time to celebrating the style and beauty of fashion models (and for good reason), in my experience, some of the chicest people in the world are behind the scenes in the fashion industry. Photographers, stylists, and the rest of the glam squad arguably have the toughest roles to fill, because while they are expected to be at the top of their style game at all times, their jobs call for them to be dressed casually so they can be on-the-go at a moment's notice. After years in the business, many of these visionaries have the casual chic look on lock. Being around this effortless-meets-polished style all the time has a major influence on many models and guides them in their own personal off-duty style. "Model off-duty" is a term industry insiders coined to describe the uncomplicated, effortless styles that models wear when they're between shoots. Their easy, relaxed vibe is matched with minimal-to-no makeup and simple but stylish accessories. This casual, cool, but put-together look resonates with me and is something I put in my work as well. The off-duty look is a major inspiration for much of my more causal designs for the RACHEL Rachel Roy collection.

THE PHILOSOPHY

There are plenty of no-fuss ways to look polished while playing the real-life role of Wonder Woman, and they don't involve sweat- or yoga pants. What you put on your body is a reflection of how you feel about yourself. It is a way to show respect to your body, your mind, and your soul as you move about your life and work. Whether you're a mother running from school to errands to the kitchen, or a young lady moving from class to work to a date, you should feel inspired by your appearance and empowered by the statement you're making. The good news is, you have so many more options than you might realize for everyday staples and put-together uniforms that can be worn with ease but still look like outfits filled with personality—your personality.

———

DASH OUT THE DOOR...

SWAP THE SWEATPANTS FOR...
Harem Pants

These loose-fitting pants feature a flexible waistband and a low crotch. Many women are fearful to wear them, because they're concerned the pants will appear unflattering or look frumpy. I encourage everyone to get over that fear, no matter what body shape or size they're working with. Harem pants can be extremely complementary and sophisticated. The key to looking good in these pants is so simple: have the ankles pegged. Creating that silhouette reminds the observer that you've got a body under all those loose layers. Finding the right fit can be daunting, yes. Try holding your arm straight downward against your leg. The material should start getting tighter from the point where the palm of your hand hits. If you find a good pair that isn't quite fitting in this way, take them to a dry cleaner or tailor. It's worth having the perfect pair around that you feel good in; they will be worn time and time again.

I hosted my daughter Tallulah's birthday party recently. I knew from experience I'd have to be dressed for a different kind of work.

There would be spills to clean up and shoelaces to tie. There would also be parents to greet and photos to pose for. I wanted to wear something uncomplicated and approachable that made me feel confident and ready for pictures that would be around for the rest of my life. I went with my harem pants and a low V-neck shirt, with a blazer and slip-on sneakers. Mission accomplished: I felt like I could be as active as I needed to be, but still polished and photo-ready.

Another trick to picking the right kind of harem pant is to consider the material: the stiffer the fabric, the better the pant will look on curvier bodies. When the fabric is thicker, it will hug your thighs less and more effectively help hide lumps and bumps. Cotton blends or wool blends are my personal favorite. Cotton blends will be our jersey substitute, and wool blends will look as polished as work wear.

Gaucho Pants

The harem pants' distant cousin the gaucho is similar in comfort but looser in structure. The thick waist-

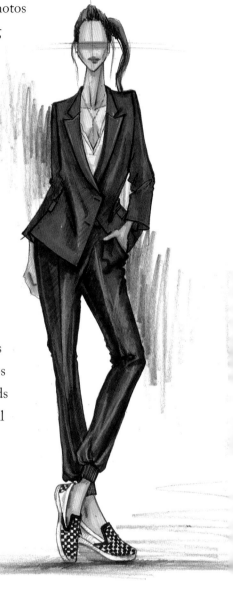

band will hug your frame, giving you flattering support that really holds you in without being suffocating. Gauchos are formal enough to wear anywhere if you style them up and accessorize correctly, but they're also comfortable enough to consider a throw-on-and-go kind of item. Long, loose wrap cardigans will break up the look and soften the overall aesthetic. And if you're having a particularly hard time giving up your yoga pant uniform or pajama-chic daywear, gauchos are the perfect option for you: they are often made from the very same fabric as yoga or even pajama pants, but they're infinitely more sophisticated and will make you feel sexy and on-trend. Why not step out in something that looks so much more put together if it's essentially the same as your less-glam staples?

Drawstring Pants

This may come as a shocker, but the very same pants I often dress down on the weekend with a turtleneck and sneakers were the exact ones I chose to wear the first time I spoke on a panel at the White House. Made of a silk-blend fabric, and finished off with a comfortable drawstring, the pants were perfect for feeling at ease and super confident. I loved that I could put my hands in my pockets while I was speaking, because it's the easiest strategy for quickly calming my nerves. I also appreciated that they were low maintenance and wouldn't need tending to if they shifted or unbuttoned, as a wrap dress might. My attention could be fully focused on what I was saying and how people were receiving me—not my outfit. The best part? These pants are basically sweatpants in a fancy fabric. A very tiny detail makes all the difference: the taut ankle cuff.

Another super-simple way to spruce up any look with drawstring pants, no matter how casual: tuck in your top to create a waistline. I wore mine with bejeweled strappy heels, a tucked-in jean shirt, and a bright magenta blazer so those in the large convention room could see me clearly. I wanted to provide insight and inspiration to my fellow women through dressing for work in an out-of-the-box manner. Thanks to some of the most powerful, influential women in the spotlight today, it has become increasingly more acceptable to dress in a more approachable style. Michelle Obama and Anna Wintour have been known to wear the same shoes or dresses multiple times—there's no false pretension that they wear an outfit once and discard it. Their message opens up a world for women to feel okay not constantly updating and upgrading their fashions, as long as they work for them. I don't need to buy or create a new dress every time I have an important event to attend. I can wear my favorite silk-blend pants and feel perfectly on point. I went onstage wanting to offer the same kind of assurance those role models have given me to other women.

THE GUIDE TO CASUAL CHIC

TOSS THE TRACKSUIT AND PUT ON . . .

A midi dress and leggings is a favorite signature outfit when I want to look polished in my off-duty time. It's also my go-to for travel. I'll wear a pair of tight leggings, which holds me in, with a long midi dress that hits between knee and ankle. The dress I choose is always made from a relaxed fabric with some stretch, which allows for a fluidity yet softness. I choose dresses that have buttons that run the length of the dress, and I'll undo them from my upper leg to create a high slit. This gives the illusion of showing leg, allowing me a youthful feel. The leggings underneath keep me from any mishaps if I'm getting out of a car or a plane and allow me to navigate busy days easily.

BYE-BYE, HOODIE, AND HELLO . . .

A sharp replacement for the sweat-shirt or jean jacket is a **leather (or faux) motorcycle jacket.** The super-lightweight ones will get more wear, as they work for various seasons. It's quite simple to style your-self with this one. Anytime you'd use a jean jacket, re-place it with this and see how it instantly elevates your outfit; plus it is just as comfortable.

When I go to the gym and it's balmy, if I need something that is not heavy but easy to grab and go—I grab my leather motorcycle jacket. It is easily thrown over dresses and trousers alike.

UNLESS YOU'RE GETTING A PEDI, LEAVE THE FLIP-FLOPS AT HOME AND . . .

Step into a pair of **laceless slip-on sneakers**. Everyone from high-price designers to fast-fashion stores is making their own version of this classic shoe. They are modern and youthful and make comfort look as it should: easy. These work seamlessly for a polished look even though you're wearing sneakers.

HANDS FREE

When it comes to traveling or just being prepared for a busy day, most of us reach for a **cross-body bag or a giant tote** to keep our hands free. You can't pack much into a cross-body, and overpacking a tote bag results in a huge bulk under your arm, making you unstable and completely defeating its purpose. Backpacks are timeless solutions to the hands-free issue.

Look for similar materials you would seek out in a handbag and hardware that is both sleek and functional.

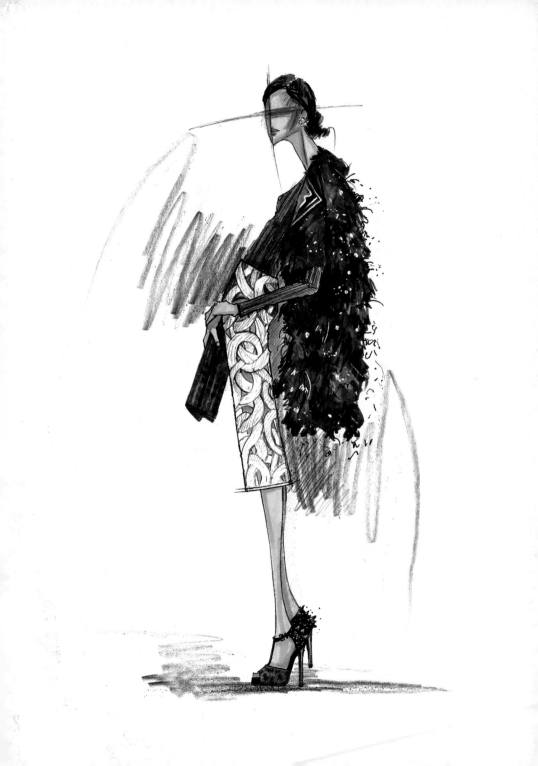

9

RUNWAY MEETS REAL LIFE

*I want everyone
to look at the
clothes and think,
"I want to be
that girl."*

—TOM FORD

R unway shows can be incredibly confusing and bewildering for many people who are not familiar with the fashion industry. Aside from the quick changes, high energy, and all-around chaos happening behind the scenes, the looks that go down the runway can sometimes be overwhelming and over-the-top, leaving those unfamiliar with the fantasy realm of fashion scratching their heads and trying to figure out who in the world could wear any of the larger-than-life looks off of the runway.

I, however, was never puzzled by how the artistry of the runway could be translated into real life. I distinctly remember when I was growing up, pouring through the pages of fashion magazines and having the directional fabrics, the pervasive color combinations, the high-octane designs, pushing me to dream. To dream a life that had zero to do with the life I was born into. Exploring fashion through magazines allowed me to imagine, to fantasize. Anything that causes you to muse and just think, to be curious, to be filled with curiosity, well, that is usually where you will find your passion. I would create stories in my head that involved what I wore in each glamour-filled twist and turn of the tale. It killed time that could have been spent being angry and confused with the household assigned to me. Instead, it allowed me to escape, as did books. So yes, the runways always made sense to me, even as a young child. They were there to inspire; they were there to create newness of thought; they were there to push forward the fashion I had access to. And that is just what they did for me. As a young girl I would daydream my odd childhood existence away with images of living abroad in inspired runway fashions. The designs I saw coming down the runway, while avant-garde, were merely gifts of thought that I made into my own wearable fashions in my head. The stories I created in my imagination got me through many tough times growing up. In large part fashion taught me to dream beyond my surroundings at a very early age. And in many ways fashion saved my life, offering me an existence beyond what I was born into because of the dream it allowed. I know this is the same for many of my friends working in fashion as well.

I tried to explain to anyone who cared that the lavish, theatrical looks and styles sometimes presented on the runway were never really intended to be worn by the average man or woman in real life. I understood quite early on that many of the runway shows were not about real life at all; in fact, the runway was meant to be a world of pure fantasy. The looks presented onstage were meant not to be interpreted literally but to serve as inspiration for real-life adaptations.

As designers we can create elaborate pieces to display in runway shows that are crafted with the intention of inspiring the audience and observers with an entirely fresh perspective and a new narrative. Whether the intent is to arouse a certain emotion, evoke the look and feel of a particular era, or motivate the audience to think critically about a particular topic or theme, we use creations to tell stories that we hope are innovative, inspirational, and sometimes completely novel. The pieces we showcase onstage serve as elements in a larger, illusory world. The extravagant items are not necessarily meant to be worn to the office, out to dinner, or while lounging around the house, although bravo to the men and women who do!

The intention behind runway shows is to always push fashion forward, and to introduce inventive and even revolutionary ideas and concepts to high-powered industry insiders and tastemakers sitting in the front row who have major influence and authority, as well as the buyers who decide what will be in the stores, and other designers who create fast fashion for the department stores based on the concepts they see. The trends and ideas born on the runway then trickle down into mainstream apparel that is meant to be not only much more affordable, but more readily wearable in everyday life. As fashion designers we know this, of course—these over-the-top looks are actually meant to inspire ideas and encourage consumers to convert trends into real life. Which is where magazines come in; they translate trends from the runway onto the pages of their publication. Bloggers have an immediate response to the runway shows, interpreting their version of what they witnessed during fashion weeks.

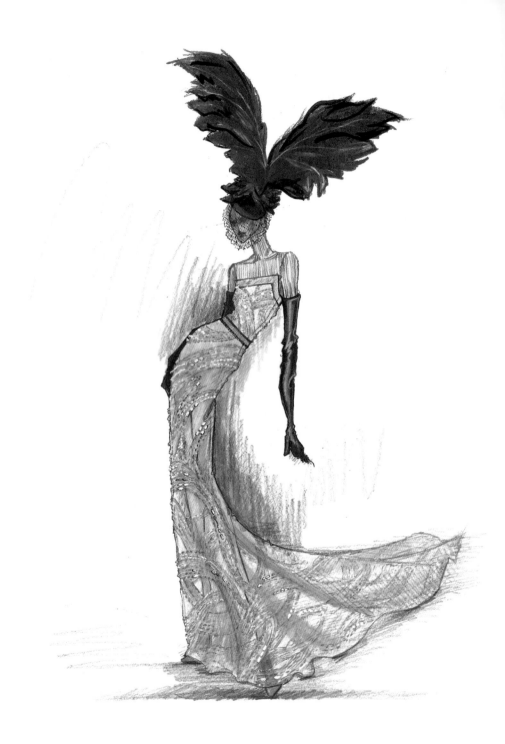

In the case of the four-foot-tall feather headdress you may see on the catwalk, you might translate that into your life by wearing a beautiful barrette in the same tone or wearing a feather-print blouse or other garment, or a tiny veiled hat decorated with just a few delicate feathers to a special event. The key is to adapt the ideas in a wearable, personalized way that isn't literal, but is fresh and different and speaks to who you are— adapting and transforming them in a way that just might add interest and richness to day-to-day outfits.

159

THE CREATION

An influential moment in my career was seeing what Tom Ford created and sent down the runway for Gucci in 1996. I was inspired watching the iconic show as model after model slithered down the runway looking effortlessly chic and donning slick menswear-influenced pieces. The overall aesthetic was both powerful and noteworthy for me. The look that solidified my love affair with menswear was a model dressed in a bloodred velvet suit paired with a white blouse unbuttoned to the navel. The look was equal parts sexy and strong, and it perfectly projected the balance of feminine and masculine that I am drawn to, admire, and try to incorporate into my own personal and professional style. The campaigns that accompanied the collection conveyed the same androgynous, unisex theme, depicting both men and women wearing the same suits and looking equally accomplished and sexy. Even Ford himself wore one of the gender-neutral shirts on the cover of *Vanity Fair*, embodying much of the same composed confidence that his models exuded on the runway and in print. The overall message through the show, the ads, and his own personal style was that despite the outdated stereotypes and conventions, women and men are in fact equal and that in order to realize their true potential for power and strength, women should not have to relinquish their femininity or sacrifice their status, self-worth, or sexuality. For me, Ford communicated this message clearly through his work, inspiring women to simultaneously embrace their femininity and softness, while feeling confident embodying the power normally reserved for men. I believe his collection was and is iconic.

The late nineties saw the rise of many powerful women in the spotlight, from musicians to movie stars to politicians. Women were rising up in the ranks and Ford's forward-thinking designs certainly reflected the cultural shift. It was an incredible statement to see take shape, and the fashion industry began to follow suit, with the proliferation of more strong, structured, but sexy shapes and silhouettes for women in the work place, where style had a new voice and new options.

THE INSPIRATION

After seeing Ford's collection and understanding the symbolism behind it and the greater context for this blending of masculine and feminine, I hoped to see more of the theme on the streets and not just on the runway. When I showed my 2006 collection a decade later, it was during a time when most designers were creating and featuring extremely hip, avant-garde, cutting-edge looks and styles. Not many were focusing on simple, beautiful, feminine classic clothes for the sophisticated working woman to wear, but that specific niche was what I was and what I have always stayed true to. Despite the fact that I was certainly in the minority and was unsure whether or not my looks would be well received, I swam against the current and pursued the passion that truly inspired me: designing for the working woman.

161

Rather than attempt to go against my natural inclination and create dark, edgy garments and accessories, I opted for the classic shapes with a twist of downtown. I focused on outfits that I felt could serve double duty between the office and an evening. Taking cues from Ford and other innovative thinkers before me, I incorporated looser, slightly baggy slacks as opposed to skintight pants, in order to give women a little room to relax and a little extra masculine attitude, which looks good on everyone. I wanted the looks to allow women to project their power and confidence out to the world, even if those qualities were still only aspirational traits they hoped to attain and didn't quite yet fully embody. I wanted women to be able to wear classic, figure-flattering pieces in fresh new ways that allowed their strength to shine through.

I will forever be happy that I did not follow the edgy trend permeating the runway and magazines at the time and decided rather to design my collection in a way that played to my strengths. This is what led to support from the fashion community; having a voice and staying authentic to it is the only path that leads to true success, in any field. Whether it's in career, relationships, family dynamics, or friendships, remaining faithfully connected to who we are, our souls, is the greatest gift we can give ourselves, our loved ones, and the larger world. Despite the dated principles and more we may have been taught to internalize, we do not have to be everything to everyone, and we do not have to sacrifice who we are in order to make others happy. We just have to be exceptional at pursuing our passions and be 100 percent authentic to ourselves in every aspect of life—**take the risk of actually being you.** It is the first risk every businessperson should take.

162

THE PHILOSOPHY

When we think of playing dress-up, we often imagine ourselves or our children digging through boxes of Halloween costumes, creating the craziest, most inventive looks and outfits imaginable, and having the most fun in the world doing it. But what happens when we grow up? Do we have to give up playing dress-up and sacrifice the fun and freedom in getting dressed up in favor of sticking to safe everyday staples that are much more "adult"? While we certainly do grow and evolve in our fashion choices, I do not believe we have to abandon the fantasy aspects of dressing up, nor do we have to let go of the idea that clothes and fashion can (and should be!) exciting. I believe getting dressed is something we should all look forward to, whether it's for a casual day or for a marathon day of meetings at the office. The difference in playing dress-up as a grown-up is learning to adapt the dreamy, unique fantasy qualities of inspirational looks to our real lifestyles and tastes. While we may not be able to literally dress from head to toe in royal robes, for example, there is no reason we can't incorporate certain elements of regal style into our everyday aesthetic. All it takes is a bit of ingenuity and willingness to explore, take risks, and enjoy the process.

GO TO THE MOVIES

Anytime I'm feeling uninspired or stuck in a style rut, I look to my favorite classic black-and-white films for inspiration. The silver-screen beauties of Old Hollywood consistently channeled a sophisticated style and attitude that line up perfectly with my own tastes. But rather than try to copycat Rita Hayworth's or Lauren Bacall's iconic wardrobes, I might try to incorporate particular elements of each lady's looks into my uniform for the day. Maybe it's by wearing a perfectly tailored pencil skirt or a figure-flattering off-the-shoulder top—I choose a few representative pieces that encapsulate

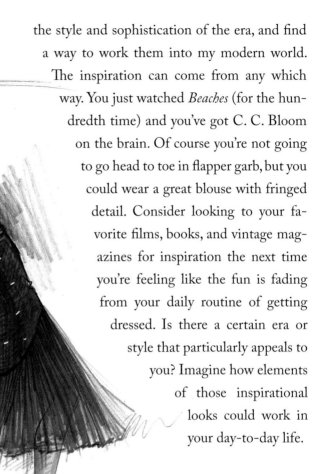

the style and sophistication of the era, and find a way to work them into my modern world. The inspiration can come from any which way. You just watched *Beaches* (for the hundredth time) and you've got C. C. Bloom on the brain. Of course you're not going to go head to toe in flapper garb, but you could wear a great blouse with fringed detail. Consider looking to your favorite films, books, and vintage magazines for inspiration the next time you're feeling like the fun is fading from your daily routine of getting dressed. Is there a certain era or style that particularly appeals to you? Imagine how elements of those inspirational looks could work in your day-to-day life.

BOOKS

Many of the literary heroines I've come to admire over the years have been independent, take-charge protagonists who are described as being just as beautiful as they are fierce. Whether these characters are from a by-gone era or are modern-day leads, I often pore over the descriptive details of their styles and pick up inspiration from the text. There is no better feeling than getting completely lost and absorbed in the story of a book. Bringing a dose of that literary adventure to every-day life can be a fun way to inject a little bit of fantasy back into the real world.

MAGAZINES

Of course, fashion magazines, the inspirational tools. These veri-table style bibles certainly contain pages of beautiful runway looks worth adapting to everyday life, but why should we limit ourselves to this particular genre of periodical? If interior design lights you up, then stock up on titles in that category and regularly look for colors, shapes, textures, and styles that appeal to your senses. If nature mag-azines speak to your interests, flip through the pages and take in the images of earth, sea, and sky, and see what ideas they evoke. Ethereal photos of clouds can translate to shades of baby blue in fabrics like chiffon. You never know where you might find fashion inspiration, and just being open to exploring outside the box and in the pages of magazines is a great way to compile ideas. It is how many designers start each collection.

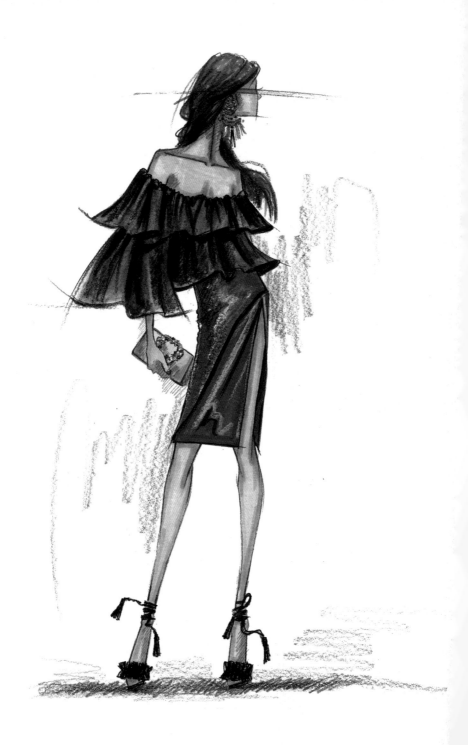

10

ALL
ABOUT
ACCESSORIES

*Give a girl
the right pair
of shoes and
she'll conquer
the world.*

—MARILYN MONROE

W e often spend so much time focusing on finding just the right garments to fill out our wardrobes that we overlook one of the most powerful ways to really elevate our style and take our looks to the next level: accessories. Although accessories can often be mistakenly seen as an afterthought, they hold real strength in their subtlety. They are the details that truly convey that a woman cares deeply about how she is perceived and who she wants to be.

Putting extra time and effort into pairing outfits with the right accessories can make all the difference between looking presentable and looking sensational.

I like to think of accessories as the tools to get me through any and all situations—whether they're planned or unexpected. If I'm not quite feeling like getting completely done up, I can downplay the dressiness of the rest of my outfit, but throw on some killer heels to completely change the look and feel of my overall style. If I don't want to go for bold allover color, but I want to stand out in a crowd, I can opt for a handbag that pops with a hint of neon or chandelier earrings that catch the light, therefore adding light to the wearer. I consider accessories my go-to style saviors that I can rely on day or night to transform my look.

Part of the reason I consider my accessories to be such tried-and-true staples is because I'm intimately familiar with the ones I own and depend on to complement my clothes. It doesn't take a separate closet full of bags and belts in order to feel prepared for any occasion. When it comes to accessories, and all areas of style for that matter, it's not the quantity that matters, but the quality and selection. This takes a bit of work up front, but by taking the time to be thoughtful and selective in choosing your accessories, you avoid having to stock up on an endless supply of bracelets, shoes, and sunglasses. The most important thing to keep in mind when amassing your accessory arsenal is to stay true to your tastes and to consider how each piece will fit into your lifestyle and complement your existing wardrobe. Referencing your vision board and putting the time and energy into finding pieces that truly speak to your style and soul will serve you well in the long run, and save you from scrambling to complete an outfit at the last minute.

It really does not take much to get caught up in the accessory game. Here is a list of accessory essentials every stylish woman should own:

LEATHER BELT, DARK BROWN

For me the best belts have a worn-in look to them, because I am usually using them to add an ease to a dressed-up outfit. For authenticity, I like finding hidden treasures at secondhand stores like Goodwill, where I tend to find surprising gems among the racks. It can take a bit of patience to seek out the perfect piece in a second-hand store, but the effort is usually well worth it. My vintage Ralph Lauren belt goes with me everywhere, and it is responsible for adding a flattering finishing touch to an array of go-to outfits. I like to wear it in both traditional and unexpected ways, cinching it over cardigans, through my jeans, or on top of a dress.

OVERSIZED CLUTCH

This simple bag is a modern, stylish option that gives off an effortless sensibility. I love any item that works double duty as a functional and fashionable piece that instantly boosts an outfit's effortless cool factor. I also love the fact that oversized clutches can be carried casually even though they have elements of elegance and opulence. I prefer to go for a neutral hue or animal print for maximum versatility, as I consider an animal print a neutral and use it in the same way.

171

CLASSIC HEELS WITH A POINTY TOE AND SINGLE SOLE

If you pay close attention to her photos, you'll see that Anna Wintour has several pairs of Manolos that she wears in rotation. While Anna could certainly switch up her shoe game every single day, never repeating the same heels twice, she knows that dependable, versatile staples are enough to transform a multitude of looks. When on the hunt for your own collection, look for classic heels without a platform to create timeless style with a denim or a pencil skirt. The single sole adds just the right amount of style and sexiness to your look, with a bit of strong, classic sophistication.

NUDE BALLET FLATS

Never underestimate the power of the perfect flat. These will take you anywhere, anytime, and go with just about anything. The neutral nude hue will add to their versatility, and the timeless style will instantly make you feel as feminine and put together as your favorite starlet from the past. They're a must-have alternative to flip-flops and other on-the-go soles that are decidedly less fashionable.

STATEMENT SHOE

In addition to classic heels, it's important to have a statement shoe for meaningful times in your life when you simply want to dress up your denim or want to completely go for a full-on high-glam moment. The style isn't set in stone; it could be a sandal, bejeweled heel, or boot. The important part is to pick something that appeals to your style and that you can see yourself building outfits around. Consider this shoe the star of the show whenever you wear it—your outfit will be the vehicle to showcase it in all its glory. The statement shoe is a special accessory that elevates your style in the same way you would elevate your overall look with statement jewelry. It speaks to who you are as a person and conveys what story you want to tell in that moment.

AVIATOR SUNGLASSES

To me, there is nothing cooler in the way of sunnies than a pair of sleek aviator shades. Not only are they undeniably fashion consistent, but, unlike other styles, they also flatter every face shape. Aviators have a hint of formalness balanced with a laid-back vibe, making them adaptable to a variety of situations and events. Aviators are my go-to and they work for just about everyone. If aviators aren't your strong suit, you can also choose a traditional-shape frame that works for your face, such as oversized round, or ones with a slight cat eye in black or tortoise—choose signature sunnies you love and then work in a few fun styles. I look for the darkest lenses. They're mysterious and protect a cosmetic-free face when in a rush, and they match almost every style of clothes so they're good to grab and go.

EVERYDAY CARRYALL TOTE

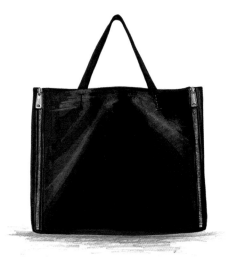

I love a structured bag, because you can basically hold your life in there and nobody has to know. That rich-looking satchel could be carrying gym clothes, but to an onlooker you likely have important papers in there instead. Hermès's Kelly bag is my inspiration for the perfect go-everywhere handbag. Look for sleek, sturdy simplicity when choosing an everyday carryall.

HARDCOVER NOTEBOOK

I always have a well-made, hardbound book with refillable paper in my bag. You never know when you'll have a sudden surge of inspiration or need to jot something down while on vacation, in a meeting,

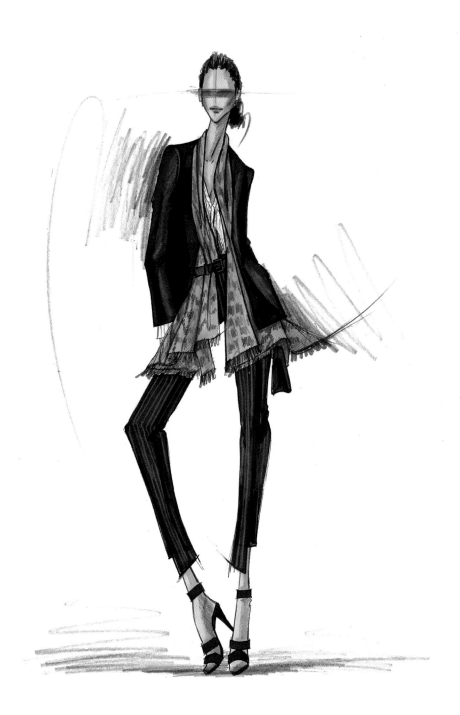

at the store, on the phone. It's smart to come prepared and it's chic to have something that looks more motivating than an old note-pad. I also keep small notepads with my initials on them—anything pleasing to the eye can serve as inspiration, and lead to great notes to better oneself!

SCARVES

Rather than thinking of scarves as an accessory reserved just for cold weather, consider them a multifunctional fashion tool. Having a va-riety of fabulous scarves can serve a host of purposes: wrapping your hair, concealing your waist and hips as a bikini cover-up, adding to a tee shirt to upscale an outfit, wrapping around the handle of your handbag for an extra bit of flair, and so on. One of my favorite ways to wear a scarf is draped over a dress or suit and tucked in beneath a belt. It adds dimension to your outfit and looks very chic. Scarves are also an easy way to work with mixed prints. Choose one that complements the pattern of one of your main pieces, and it will take your ensemble to the next level of style.

175

BRIGHT LIPSTICK

As with fashion, always select makeup shades that work best for your skin tone and hair color. A great, rich pigment on your lips is a pleasant mood booster and an instant outfit upgrader. I al-ways have a Nars pencil lipstick in Dragon Girl on hand, just in case!

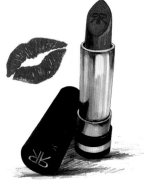

PERSONALIZED STATEMENT JEWELRY

Long ago, I purchased a beautiful Bea Valdes necklace handmade in the Philippines from natural stones. No matter how mundane or ordinary my outfit, the necklace makes a grand statement. There are so many elements that make me feel special when I wear it. The natural stones make me feel grounded, it is unique and unlike anything anyone else usually has on, and a female designer whom I respect designed it. Whether it's earrings from a loved one, a bracelet someone made you, or a ring you bought on a celebration day, your personal piece should uplift you, taking you to a place that makes you feel happy. Elle Macpherson wears an armful of arm candy, always—pieces she has collected from her travels. Fashion's global icon, Carine Roitfeld, wears a long chain adorned with charms from her friends and family. Once when I was shopping at Fred Leighton with André Leon Talley, we saw a charm bracelet formerly owned by Marlene Dietrich. Each charm was engraved with a quote from a lover of hers. It really doesn't get much more personal than that! The more personal the piece, the better, because it is a reflection of you and what you love.

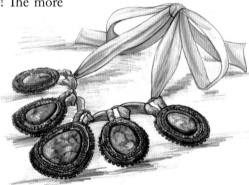

· CONCLUSION ·

EXPERIENCE
AND
INNOCENCE

Love yourself first
and everything else
falls into line.
You really have to
love yourself to
get anything done
in this world.

—LUCILLE BALL

One of the most transformative experiences of my life occurred when I was sixteen and went to visit my uncle and aunt who were missionaries in Mali at the time.

My uncle George worked with the government on ways to improve the economic conditions there through an initiative their church conference headed up; and, as Mali is a French-speaking country, my aunt Ellen interpreted all the French legal documents for the programs that were developed. George and Ellen had been there for quite a few years before my family had the opportunity to visit them, and even though I knew it would be a tough trip, as all third world trips can be, it was a highly anticipated journey, to say the least. My parents never had a lot of money but they always found ways to make sure we saw as much of the world as we could, which was my mother's intent when she planned the trip for my brother and me—to experience the world. And experience it we did, starting from the floor of the food tent in the village we were visiting. That's where my mother, brother, and I had to sleep. The tent housed bags of grain dropped from the sky by the Red Cross and similar organizations. They were intended to feed the small village, but they also proved a big draw for local vermin. While the rats running over my hair and feet as we "slept" on the floor were so horrid it was hard to believe it was really happening, the real nightmare was the spiders, which I swear were the size of small babies and lived in the one outdoor toilet the village had set up for our use. For me, what this meant was that I would not be going to the bathroom for the four days that we were there—yes, dying from within was preferable to the thought of getting bitten by one of those otherworldly, deadly monsters. Spiders to this day are one of my biggest phobias.

What kept me going during that emotionally difficult trip was what I learned through observation. When we arrived after days of traveling, the children ran alongside the truck as we drove in, swarming us with hugs, smiles, and greetings that I could not understand. A group of girls, ranging in age from two to twenty, hung on my arms and my every movement from the minute I stepped out of the truck. They wanted to see everything I had brought with me, but the thing they were most interested in was my makeup. Who knows what possessed me, at age sixteen, to bring cosmetics to the middle of the desert, but I suppose that everything does happen for a reason. My lip balms, lipsticks, compacts, and perfumes were most certainly not on the list of carefully thought-out and useful items my aunt and uncle advised us to bring. But they were just part of me and worth the effort, despite the extra space they took up and the fact that they were halfway melted by the time we arrived.

What I could not have imagined, however, was the delight I witnessed when those girls discovered my makeup, put it on, and looked at their reflection, many for the first time ever seeing themselves outside of their reflection in water; it was life-changing. The pure joy that their made-up reflections gave them not only provided us a common ground that I shared with them uniquely apart from my mother and brother, but also showed me that little girls are little girls no matter where they are from and what they are born into; and that fashion, makeup, and accessories can bring so much pure happiness to people. This is the part of the fashion and beauty industry that I adore. I was so moved by how those girls loved themselves, how they loved their reflections, and that is key: loving yourself. Once that falls into place it opens a world of endless opportunities to create happiness within. The juxtaposition of what I was experiencing—my fears and phobias coming to life versus the simple but profound joy getting made up gave those girls—was important in shaping who I am as a person. Beauty is all around, even when you are scared or feel lost, alone, or misunderstood. By wearing what I loved literally on my sleeve, I quickly met like-minded souls and we bonded much more quickly than my mother or brother bonded with the villagers. I had found my tribe, girls who liked to laugh, play with makeup, and just be girls. Of course, this is not the only way to cross barriers, but it certainly is a universal truth that what makes us smile will make our friends and those with similar ideals smile, too. I found my people within moments of arriving and my connection with them made dealing with my fears pale in comparison.

This lesson about loving yourself and finding joy, however you can and no matter the circumstances, is something I've carried with me ever since, and something I continually seek to imbue my work with. Every day I strive to help women gain self-confidence and awareness of their own unique beauty and the qualities that make them special.

I have gone back to Africa several times since then, each time learning something more about myself. At the core of that first trip I learned the value of joy. It is priceless and yet it is free. And it is our responsibility to discover what brings us joy. When I get stuck emotionally or creatively, as is easy to do, I reference my vision/mood board as a visual reminder of what makes me happy. I also try to reflect outward, and do something for someone else that gets me from zero to joy in no time flat.

INSPIRING EACH OTHER

One day, my elder daughter returned home from the elementary school she attended right outside of New York City and insisted we go shopping in SoHo for a specific trending outfit that would help her fit in with the other girls at school. I knew I had a quick decision to make as a mother. Certainly we've all wanted to feel accepted at different points in our lives, especially in school, but I knew this was a significant opportunity that I could use as a teaching moment. I wanted my daughter to understand that it was more important to have her own style, her own voice, than to concern herself with what others were thinking, doing, wearing, or saying. I didn't want to unfairly deny her the chance to feel solidarity with her friends and classmates, but my desire to teach her a valuable lesson was far more pressing than any guilt I had about depriving her of a trendy outfit. And so she threw a fit as we walked past the downtown store without buying the trendy tracksuit she so badly wanted. The next school day I dressed her in mismatched earrings and two different shoes that actually matched in a really cute, Carrie Bradshaw way. Ava did not want to be an experiment and gave me a tremendous amount of attitude, but I promised her that this outfit would create trends and that her friends would be copying her within the next two weeks. If they did not, I vowed that I would buy her whatever tracksuit she wanted. We had a deal.

Not long after Ava's meltdown over velour, I had a red carpet movie premiere to attend. I knew there would be a crowd of photographers there, and of course I wanted to look my best. However, rather than selecting a conventional red carpet look, I opted for something far less predictable, yet far more in line with my mood at the time. I walked the carpet in silk, pinstriped pajamas with heels and an oversized soft clutch, and felt confident in the unusual ensemble choice. When I returned home that night, I did exactly what most people in the public eye try desperately to avoid: I sat the girls down in front of the computer and dug up all the Internet comments piling up about my outfit. We scrolled through tweets and tabloid commentary, and let's just say some of the reviews were less than raves! The initial sting of the negative comments was quickly quelled by the knowledge and determination I had that I loved what I wore that night, and felt good in it, and, more important, I felt like *me* in it.

Not only did I want my daughters to see that I'd intentionally opted to go off the beaten path with my outfit in order to do what felt great to me that night, but I wanted them to see me laughing at what the online "critics" had to say and the ease with which I dismissed their negative reviews. I wanted them to understand that being true to yourself is the first step to true happiness, and I wanted them to see I was willing to actually take the risk without worrying about someone else's opinion of me. I wanted them to understand that trying to please everyone—and really, trying to please *anyone*—is a losing battle; an unnecessary, stress-inducing way to go through life. You have no control over what people think and feel, and the best thing you can do in your style, actions, and intentions is to do what works for you and feels beautiful. Because the truth is, if you make yourself happy, that's good enough and will inspire more than you ever know.

I also wanted my girls to see that if I was going to make one of them take what must have felt like an enormous risk for a little girl by going to school in a mismatched outfit, her mother was right by her side doing the same thing in public. Needless to say, the girls at Ava's private school copied her within days, because all they needed was the inspiration to be different. Most of us do. Lesson learned. Today I have a confident teenager who looks people in the eye when talking to them, wears mismatched earrings, speaks up for what she knows to be right, and defends her friends when they are picked on.

There is so much we want to get done in this lifetime, and if there's one lesson I want most to pass on, one thing that I wish I had learned at an earlier age, it's that *you* are in control. Your choices are yours to make. Whether it's where you live, what you wear, or who and what you surround yourself with, each choice the universe presents you with is a chance to create your own path. Make meaningful ones that change the quality of life for yourself and those that you love. We can design the lives we wish to live, one decision, one choice, at a time.

CARE FOR
WHAT YOU LOVE

One of my many duties in my first job as stock girl at Contempo Casuals was to prepare clothes coming in from the warehouse for the sales floor.

The pieces would arrive tightly packed in hefty boxes and had to be brought back to life in order to look presentable to shoppers. Right out of the box, the items usually didn't strike me as covetable must-haves. They were stiff, smelled from the boxes or factory life, and were wrinkled from shipping; they did not have much appeal at all. However, once I hung them on a hanger and diligently steamed them into their intended state, they somehow transformed into items we all were lusting over. It was a lesson that stayed with me always: taking proper care of clothing and accessories can make a world of difference. The little details involved in carefully maintaining the look of your items can take them from dapper to drab, and all it takes is a little effort. My work responsibilities began bleeding over into my personal time as I began paying special attention to my own closet. Like many people just starting out in their first jobs, I didn't have much money but still wanted to own nice things, or, at the very least, I wanted my things to look luxe. I've always felt that when I make an investment in something large or small, I want my things to not only last as long as possible, but also look their most beautiful after many, many uses. This means laundering items properly, treating them kindly, and keeping them in pristine condition throughout their shelf life. I know hunting down the right hangers and seeking out the right steamer can seem so tedious, boring, and time-consuming. The thing is, investing the extra moments in doing these things now will save you time in the long run. To this day, I am able to wear the designer shoes I saved up for in college because they are still in noteworthy shape. I've seen firsthand how incredible it is what a little extra love and care can do to bring new life to the belongings you already have.

Here are the tips and tricks from the people I admire most—whom I turn to for advice on everything from how to keep clothes wrinkle-free to the secrets of creative tailoring, to the power of the perfect bra—for getting your clothes and accessories to look their absolute best, so that they properly represent the ambitious attitude you want to project to the world.

RR'S TRICKS OF THE TRADE

HOW TO KEEP BELOVED BELONGINGS LOOKING THEIR ABSOLUTE BEST: STEAMERS VS. IRONS

I am a true believer in steamers when it comes to caring for clothes. When steamed, clothes look the way they're meant to because they hang the way they're meant to drape on your body—as opposed to being flattened and pressed against an ironing board. In my years of working in retail stores, we would always steam the clothes in the back room before they hit the floor. It's no different now that I'm a designer: in our sample rooms and backstage at runway shows, we also use steam. It's simply the best tool for changing the look of the clothing 100 percent and breathing life into limp, listless garments. It is quick, easy, and not as expensive as one might assume. I even travel with a mini portable steamer, which is a lifesaver in terms of both expense and time.

If you do use an iron, always use the lowest setting and follow the instructions on your clothing. Go slowly, as rushing will always lead to a burn in your clothing or, worse, on you. I have the scar on my thigh to prove it. Now if I have somewhere to go and steaming isn't an option, I make a huge effort to do it well ahead of time.

HOW TO PROTECT AND CARE FOR YOUR SHOES, WHETHER THEY COST YOU $15.99 OR $1,599

My first big "investment" item—remember those Manolos I bought on-sale when I was twenty-two—made me feel exquisitely rich in taste, which was a feeling I certainly wasn't familiar with experiencing at that age. I had saved and saved, and also made friends with the shoe salesman at Neiman Marcus in the mall where I worked. Despite a tiny twinge of guilt when I pocketed the receipt afterward, I never looked back. Quality rarely fades if you treat investment pieces like a treasure, as I did. There are plenty of ways to preserve the beauty and wearability of good-quality shoes like those classic Manolos. Adding a thin rubber sole makes shoes infinitely more comfortable, and it extends the life of your investment heels. Those rubber sole-savers come in a variety of colors and blend right in with the bottom of the shoe. Red, black, beige, white—this small but oh-so-worth-it investment will be just one of the reasons you will be the last lady standing—literally. When I lived in New York, I swore by the shoe experts at Leather Spa, a veritable haven for all damaged, distressed, and otherwise in-need-of-some-love leather accessories. I always felt safe and secure bringing my best pieces there because the staff is trained in repairing and caring for the most well-known and delicate luxury brands. I definitely encourage you to seek out a similar service in your area, but if you can't find one that meets this level of quality in your own city, Leather Spa accepts mail-in orders. So worth it!

There's a good reason shoes deserve so much attention and care: they are without a doubt the hardest-working items in your closet. If you've spent a winter in New York City—or in any city with a cold, harsh climate—you know what I'm talking about. Your shoes trudge through snow, sleet, and sludge, then get drinks spilled on them as they get stepped on at crowded soirees. We think of shoes primarily from an aesthetic point of view, as something that can instantly alter the appearance of an outfit, taking it from casual to cocktail-ready in seconds, but they also go through war on a daily basis. Which is one more reason they deserve all the tender loving care you can offer in the form of careful maintenance.

I always make a point to return my shoes to the shelf, or the shoebox, looking just the way they did when I took them out. A theory in life that I subscribe to is that we should always leave people happier or lighter than when we found them. The same theory goes for my shoes. Clean them gently with a soft cloth, especially if they're made of a delicate material. If they're suede, using a suede brush regularly will keep them looking as close to new as possible. I keep both a soft brush and a soft cloth in the same area as my shoes to make it easy to do. Seriously, two minutes on each shoe makes a world of difference. Also be sure to use the right type of storage material—for example, tall, soft boots need something sturdy inside them (tissue or newspaper is an inexpensive and effective option) to help them stand up straight so they don't end up flopped over on their sides, worn and wrinkled.

We all go through shoe phases where we find ourselves wearing our favorite shoe of thc week, the month, or maybe even the season. It can be hard to put the perfect pair of heels away when you feel like you've hit the jackpot in terms of style, comfort, and versatility. However, just like a bra, shoes need a break. It's best not to wear the same pair every single day, so switching them out every two days or so can give them time to breathe, reshape, and recover from the hot summer sun or the wintry salted ground. Give your shoes this extra bit of love and they'll continue to love you back for much longer than they would otherwise.

THE ONE THING YOU CAN'T SKIP OUT ON

I happen to be quite tall—just over five feet ten—and of course have girlfriends ranging in height from very petite to very tall, and yet, somehow, we all shop for the same jeans, from the same racks. Designer jeans are notoriously designed for the long-limbed, and the reality is that many of us just don't need so much fabric from the knee down. If only I could tack the business card of my tailor to the racks in these stores to tell every woman that her life—or at least her legs and tush—could be even better if she'd just tailor the denim to fit her to a T.

A good tailor will be your new best friend. That dress that you favor, but that just bunches strangely at the hips? Fixable. Those jeans that are getting ragged under your heels? Fixable. That beautiful blazer you sprung for that won't button over your bust? Fixable. All of these wardrobe snafus are 100 percent fixable if you can just find a great tailor. And use that tailor over and over and over again. It can seem daunting to seek out professional tailoring on a pricey item you already feel like you invested good money in, but the truth is, spending the extra time and dollars to tailor a wonderful, timeless piece that you adore will be far cheaper than replacing it annually with a cheap, ill-fitting substitute that never feels good when you put it on. I cannot emphasize this enough—a perfectly tailored pair of pants is one of the great luxuries of this world, and once you discover this for yourself, you'll wonder how you got along for so many years without the help of a tailor. Trust me on this: a talented tailor will change your life. It may be much easier to find this lifesaver than you think—I found my first one in my local dry cleaner.

THE BEAUTY OF THE BRA

This one is major: many women don't understand the infinite difference the right bra can make with any outfit. Certain bras are meant to make specific styles look better, and the shape of your bra and how it enhances the shape of your chest once in the bra can completely change the look of your outfit and even impact your posture and confidence.

Do yourself a huge favor and go to a proper bra store at least once in your life. Get fitted by a professional, and have her choose bras that are the right fit for your unique shape and body. The bras most of us are wearing are completely wrong for our breast size and type, and do nothing to flatter, shape, enhance, or otherwise help our overall appearance. Been there, done that—and what a difference once I knew my correct size. This might prove to be one of the most useful hours of shopping you've ever spent.

When it comes to different styles of bras, think about what kind of look you're going for. If you're going for hippie bohemian, opt for a bra that has less structure, no underwire. You won't achieve the loose and free-spirited look if you have a firm and lifted brassiere. If you are large busted and want the hippie chic look and can't go underwire free, then opt for a deep V shape that separates your chest to the point that your breasts are not touching and are separated by at least a few inches.

Likewise, when you're wearing a top with a deep V or an unbuttoned blouse, look for a bra that separates and elongates your chest, rather than one that creates more cleavage. It's very slenderizing and youthful. Otherwise, in push-up bras, you'll have a Victorian look, which is unflattering and very dated.

THE CLOSET

The relationship I have with my closet has always depended greatly on the condition I keep it in. It's so easy to let things get out of control, to shut the door and hide the mess. I know that when my closet is chaotic I feel less confident in its contents. That dreaded feeling of "I have nothing to wear" may seem like it's rooted in fact, but it usually stems from the anxiety created by an unorganized scene. It was my dear friend Linda Rothschild, professional closet organizer and creator of Cross It Off Your List, who taught me how to design my space not only in a way that would save me time and create order, but also in a way that would help me best care for my investments, and keep them looking their best.

When I keep my closet orderly and neat, not letting it slip too far, picking out my clothes on any given day will be a calm and inspired ritual, rather than the first battle in the war that is my busy day. I strive for my clothes, and my life, to be under my control, not subject to total chaos. And when I stay on top of this, I'm able to find what I need, look the way I want to look, and project the image of that woman I aspire to be; it is one less thing to have to deal with during a busy day of balancing. These are the tips that keep my closet as ordered and peaceful as we all wish our lives would be.

Tips from Linda Rothschild

Blazers should be on a shaped hanger rather than a very skinny hanger. Think of the shape of your shoulder—they may take up more closet space, but it's worth it to keep them in good condition.

Organizing your closet by category makes choosing outfits easier. Picture your pants hanging with pants and your skirts with skirts. You will be able to see what you have and might even wear more of your clothes. Within each category, organize by color—hanging light to dark. Not only will it be easier to find what you are looking for, but your closet will also inspire you to make outfits you may not have thought of before.

One of the biggest mistakes is not using all the space in the closet. There is often hidden and underused space lost by not being organized. Make your closet user-friendly. Hanging clothes by length reveals space you didn't know you had. When all your tops are together, for example, it frees up space underneath for shoe cubbies or a chest of drawers. Space on the top of the closet is often lost

because there's only one lonely shelf above the bar. Adding another shelf gives you additional space for boxes of out-of-season clothes or things you don't need to get your hands on all the time, freeing the space on the first shelf for folded jeans or workout clothes that are in regular rotation.

Edit, edit, edit! Beyond having everything sorted into categories, really look at each piece and try on the ones you need to. If you love it but it doesn't love you, it doesn't belong in your closet. You may love that mohair sweater, but if every time you put it on you take it off because it itches, does it really need to take up space? We all go through it—everyone makes shopping mistakes and our bodies, styles, and lifestyles change. Be realistic about what works and what you will never wear again. Be selective about what lives in your closet.

We need several types of hangers to manage our wardrobes. Although slim velvet hangers are all the rage, use them selectively. They take up the least amount of space, which is why they are so popular, but that means you're squishing in the maximum amount of clothes, which isn't always best for the clothes. They are good for certain tops and dresses but not for everything. Jackets, heavy cardigans, and coats need hangers with a little wider shoulder. Pants, depending on how much space you have, can long hang on a hanger with clips or hang short on a hanger with a bar they fold over. Try to stay away from men's bulky wood hangers—they are usually too big for women's clothes and there are so many better options. Whatever you choose, keep them consistent—it's amazing how much more organized your closet looks when all the hangers are coordinated.

The hardest part of organizing is making the decision to keep it or let it go, not what pretty containers to buy. Be honest about what you're keeping and why. Do you have the space? Does it make sense that you're keeping this? Are you really ever going to use it again? Does it make you smile? Keep things for the right reasons and in the right places.

Organize in small bites. Start with a drawer or a shelf. If you're sorting books or socks, look at everything one by one and make the decision—keep, toss, donate. It may take ten minutes or two hours, but you will feel a sense of accomplishment when it's done. If you overwhelm yourself with big projects, you'll quickly get discouraged and think you'll never get them done. Organizing can be a very cleansing and rewarding experience if you approach it the right way.

Start every day from an organized place. Be clear about where you are going, what you need to take with you, what you need to get done, and how much time you have to manage. Have realistic expectations of what can get done in a day. We all have twenty-four hours, and having good time-management skills helps us use our time more effectively. Good list-making can be critical to staying organized. Writing things down helps your head be clear instead of cluttered with everything you're trying to remember to do.

Being organized is something that doesn't come naturally to everyone. For some people it means having everything perfectly contained and labeled and put away, but that's not always attainable; nor does it have to be. Finding your keys, paying your bills on time, being able to find the shoes you want to wear, and having friends and family come to visit anytime without your being embarrassed are all attainable. Being organized can affect every part of your life from your home to your office to your relationships. You're able to find things easily without sifting through a lot of items that are in the wrong place. You have simple systems for processing mail and papers and things that ended up in a pile before because you didn't know what else to do with them. You have more of a sense of control over your environment versus feeling your things have control over you. You always save time and money—on so many levels. But organizing is not something you do once and it goes away. The clothes don't jump on the hangers themselves. You have to incorporate organizing into your daily routine.

Organizing can make a difference in other people's lives, too. It helps when making decisions to know you're not throwing things in the trash—there is someone out there who needs this or wants this more than you. Anything that's usable—from household items to clothing—can be passed along. Whatever you've decided doesn't need to be in your life any longer will make someone else happy. Donate to charity—every town has thrift stores and community bazaars and local people who need help getting back on their feet. Or have a tag sale, give things to your family, or have a swap party with your friends. Just keep it moving.

ACKNOWLEDGMENTS

There are a vast number of people in my life—
past and present—who have helped shape who I
am today and continue to contribute to who I will
become. These are people who have celebrated
my life's successes and challenges and have
always believed in me. For that I am grateful and
hope to give back to you, all that you have given
to me. All of my gratitude and love to you.

HarperCollins books may be purchased for educational, business, or sales promotional use. For information please e-mail the Special Markets Department at SPsales@harpercollins.com.

FIRST EDITION

Literary Agent: Kirsten Neuhaus
Editor: Denise Oswald
Illustrations: Soyeon Kwon
Page design: Ashley Tucker
Cover design: Mumtaz Mustafa
Publicity: Katie Steinberg
Marketing: Kendra Newton

Library of Congress Cataloging-in-Publication Data has been applied for.

ISBN 978-0-06-240512-8

16 17 18 19 20 OV/QGT 10 9 8 7 6 5 4 3 2 1